SPINE SURGERY

Edited by **Kook Jin Chung**

Spine Surgery
Edited by Kook Jin Chung

Published by InTech
Janeza Trdine 9, 51000 Rijeka, Croatia

Publishing Process Manager Sandra Bakic

Technical Editor Teodora Smiljanic

Cover Designer InTech Design Team

Additional hard copies can be obtained from orders@intechopen.com

Spine Surgery, Edited by Kook Jin Chung
p. cm.
ISBN 978-953-51-0469-8

For EU product safety concerns:
IN TECH d.o.o., Prolaz Marije Krucifikse Kozulić 3, 51000 Rijeka, Croatia,
info@intechopen.com or visit our website at intechopen.com.

Meet the editor

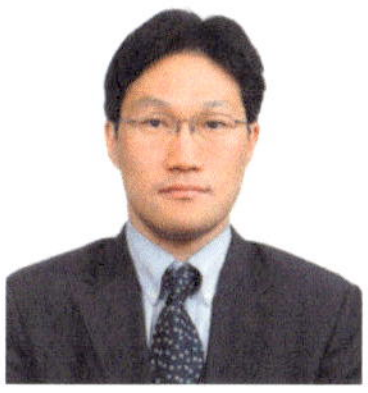

Dr Kook Jin Chung specializes in spine surgery, osteoporosis, as well as orthopaedic basic science. Dr. Chung is currently Chair for Spine Center in Kangnam Sacred Heart Hospital, Hallym University Medical Center and an Associate Professor of Orthopaedic Surgery in Hallym University. He conducts both clinical and translational studies on spinal disorders, osteoporosis and orthopaedic basic science. He is an prolific writer and also an active participant in the peer review process for several international journals in the field of orthopaedic surgery.

Contents

Preface

"Spine Surgery" is an authoritative and didactic textbook on the various fields of spine.

It is written by many authors, internationally honorable experts to share their opinions with you.

The chapters cover from anatomy of spine, spinal imaging technique, biology of spine, bone graft substitute, minimally invasive spinal surgery to even spinal deformity.

It has many up to date results to help readers including university graduate students, medical instrumentation developers, and medical professionals including orthopaedic and neurosurgeons, rehabilitative professionals.

The readers are provided with precious information and valuable guide in your daily practice.

Dr. Kook Jin Chung
Department of Orthopedic Surgery,
Kangnam Sacred Heart Hospital,
College of Medicine, Hallym University,
South Korea

Part 1

Osteoporotic Vertebral Compression Fractures

1

Unilateral Transpedicular Balloon Kyphoplasty for the Osteoporotic Vertebral Compression Fracture

Kyoung-Suok Cho and Sang-Bok Lee
Uijongbu St. Mary's Hospital, The Catholic University School of Medicine
Korea

1. Introduction

The National Osteoporosis Foundation has estimated that more than 100 million people worldwide are at a risk for the development of fractures secondary to osteoporosis.[15, 16]

Osteoporotic Vertebral compression fractures (OVCFs) constitute a major health care problem in western countries, not only because of the high incidence of these lesions but also due to their direct and indirect negative consequences for patient health-related quality of life and the costs to the health care system. Compression fractures lead to a loss of height of the vertebral segment, and the resulting spinal deformity can lead to a decrease in pulmonary capacity, malnutrition, decreased mobility, and depression. Kyphosis secondary to osteoporotic vertebral compression fractures is associated with a 2 to 3 times greater incidence of death due to pulmonary causes.[5,11,13,17]

Although usual treatment of an osteoporotic vertebral compression fracture consists of bed rest, analgesics, and bracing, some fractures go on to progressive deformity and debilitating pain.

Vertebroplasty (VP) and kyphoplasty (KP) are not only relatively simple procedures, but also less traumatic procedures for OVCF as compared to extensive stabilization surgery. Several techniques have been developed for simpler and safer procedures during the last 2 decades. Techniques of vertebral body augmentation have been developed in an effort to treat these refractory cases. The high-pressure injection of low viscosity of polymethylmethacrylate(PMMA) has potential risk for neural compromise and pulmonary embolism by uncontrolled leakage. Therefore, balloon kyphoplasty and vertebroplasty using a large cannula low-pressure injection of PMMA in a high viscosity state (so called osteoplasty) has been introduced. Percutaneous kypoplasty (PKP) is a recently developed, minimally invasive surgical treatment for OVCF. It is designed to address the fracture-related pain and the associated spinal deformity (figure 1). PKP with acrylic cement (PMMA) is a procedure aimed at preventing vertebral body collapse and pain in patients with pathologic vertebral bodies. PKP is a promising therapeutic technique for pain control in patients with bone failure. PKP for OVCFs is typically performed by delivering double balloons via a bilateral transpedicular approach, and both balloons are inflated simultaneously for elevating the end plate for accompanying vertebral body height balanced restoration. The deformity is purportedly corrected by the insertion and expansion of a balloon in a fractured vertebral body. After reduction of the fracture bone, cement is then deposited into the cavity created by the balloon to repair the fracture. Good clinical outcomes as well as restoration of vertebral body height have been reported with kyphoplasty.[3,9,12]

The unilateral single balloon technique (via the unipedicular or extrapedicular route) has been developed (Fig. 1A, B). This technique reduces trauma to the patient, procedure time, costs and radiation exposure of a patient and an operator. In particular, the needle traverses a short distance of the bony structure in the extrapedicular approach, therefore, this approach causes less pain as compared to transpedicular approach and can avoid the sclerotic area of the vertebra. In the literature, there exists a detailed anatomical understanding at the thoracic level, but not the lumbar level. Theoretically, an alternative unipedicular approach would reduce by 50% the risk associated with cannulation of the pedicles, while also reducing operative time, radiation exposure, and costs. There is some technical report about the unilateral transpedicular approach, but limited data about the effects of unilateral transpedicular kyphoplasty on clinical and radiological outcome in large patients group is available. The purpose of this chapter to describe the performance of a procedure known as inflatable bone tamp via a unilateral transpedicular approach and determine the efficacy of unipedicular transpedicular approach and the clinical and radiological outcomes.

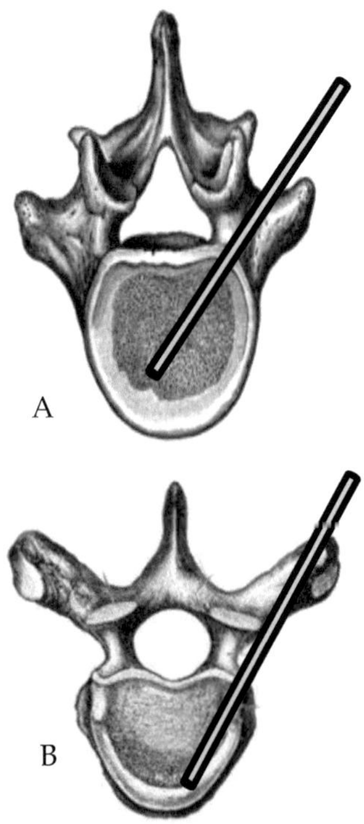

Fig. 1. Drawings views demonstrate the transpedicular approach (A) in lumbar vertebra and extrapedicular approach (B) in thoracic vertebra.

2. Principle

The analgesic effect of cement cannot be explained by the consolidation of pathologic bone alone (Fig 2). The origin of the pain in a patient with vertebral benign or malignant collapse or fracture is mostly related to the stretching of the periosteal fibers or nervous structures compression with transmission of the pain to the paravertebral nervous plexus, through the nerve ganglion and spinothalamic-parietal-cortical tract. In fact, good pain relief is obtained after injection of only 2 mL of PMMA in metastases. In these cases, the consolidation effect is minimal. The methylmethacrylate is cytotoxic because of its chemical and thermal effects during polymerization. The temperature during polymerization is high enough to produce coagulation of tumoral cells. Therefore, good pain relief can be obtained with a small volume of cement.

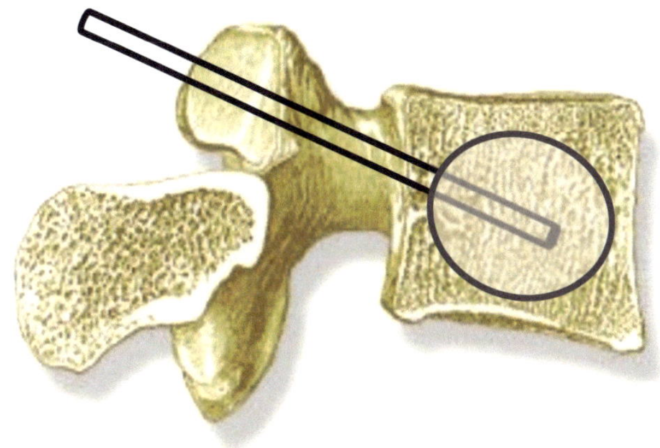

Fig. 2. Drawing demonstrates the principle of percutaneous cementoplasty at the lumbar level, showing vertebral puncture via the posterolateral route and vertebral filling.

3. Inclusion criteria

Clinical indications for kyphoplasty should be based on a detailed medical history and careful examination of the patient. Patients with acute spine thoracic or lumbar pain generally refer to a physician that, after a clinical evaluation, will suggest a medical therapy and a short-term follow-up. If the back pain does not decrease, physician should be performed radiograph examinations to find normal findings or the presence of an initial vertebral fracture. After at least 4 to 6 weeks from the beginning of clinical symptomatology, if the pain does not subside in spite of maximum medical treatment, MRI evaluation is suggested to distinguish between benign versus malignant are well known, but sometimes differential diagnosis is not simple, especially in cases of vertebral fracture related to multiple myeloma. In patients with metastatic disease, a bone scan is useful for a systemic oncological balance. However, many patients have multiple fractures and lack sufficient imaging studies to document the age of some or all of the fractures. Others have several adjacent fractures in which it is difficult to determine, by physical examination, the fracture that is symptomatic. In such instances, magnetic resonance (MR) imaging with gadollium enhancement is helpful, with edema within the marrow space of the vertebral body best visualized on sagittal T2-weighted images. Bone scans can be used to help differentiate the symptomatic level from incidentally discovered fractures. The ideal candidate for kyphoplasty presents within 3 months of fracture and has midline, non-radiating back pain that increases with weight bearing and can be exacerbated by manual palpation of the spinous process of the involved vertebra. Selection criteria for kyphoplasty were described in Table 1.

3.1 Contraindications

1. Hemorrhagic diathesis.
2. Infection.
3. Lesions with epidural extension. These require careful injection to prevent epidural overflow and spinal cord compression by the cement or displaced epidural tissue.

The absolute contraindications are the presence of local or systemic infections, the presence of an epidural or foraminal extension associated with neurologic deficit and uncorrectable coagulation disorders. Vertebra plana, mixed secondary lesion, disruption, or epidural extension of the posterior vertebral wall are relative contraindications related to physician's experience in most cases.

Indications
Vertebral fracture pain
Sufficient pain to impair activities of daily living
Failure of reasonable medical therapy and time
Comprehensive medical evaluation of osteoporotic vertebral compression fractures
Technical feasibility
Sufficient medical stability to tolerate general anesthesia
Absence of contraindication
Contraindications
Hemorrhagic diathesis
Infection
Lesions with epidural extension

Table 1. Indication for Unilateral transpedicular balloon kyphoplasty.

4. Operative technique

The operative procedure was performed under aseptic conditions in an operating room while blood pressure, heart rate, electrocardiography, and pulse oximetry parameters were continuously monitored. Before the procedures, 25 mg of Demerol was injected intravenously to control pain. Percutaneous kyphophoplasty was performed using fluoroscope via a unilateral transpedicular approach. Usually, a right-handed operator stood on the left side of a patient for a left-side approach. PKP must be performed in sterile conditions and intravenous antibiotics are generally administrated few hours before the procedure. In most cases, local anesthesia can be administered by injection (ie, 2 to 3 mL of 2% lidocaine hydrochloride) at the skin level and deeper, to include the periosteum, with a 22-gauge spinal needle. Occasionally, conscious sedation can be useful for uncooperative patients or in poor clinical conditions. After conscious sedation and the patient was carefully positioned prone on the fluoroscopy table. The authors recommended targeting the tip of a needle in the vertebra was in the mid-line and anterior one-third of the vertebra body for vertebroplasty and in the center of the body for balloon kyphoplsty (Fig. 3).

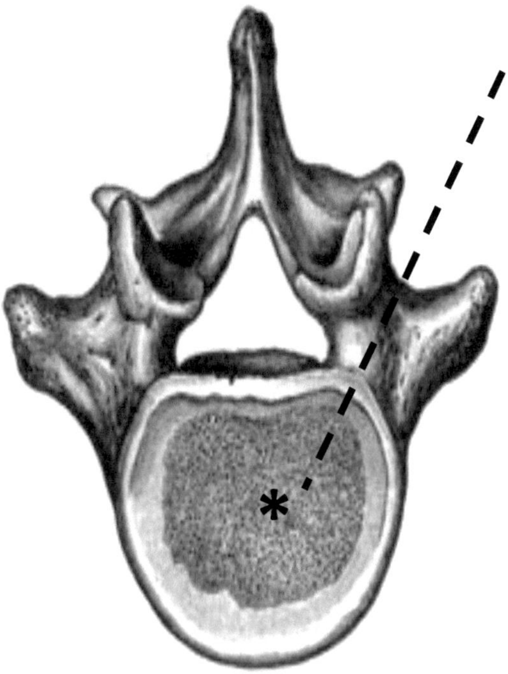

Fig. 3. In the lower lumbar area, the lateral wall of the pedicle (dotted line) can be used for an entry point due to the greater width of the lower lumbar pedicle. (* target point).

The trajectory line was made between the target point of the needle tip and the skin entry point through the transverse process (TP). Once the skin incision for the entry point was made, adjusting the direction of the needle was limited due to large lumbar dorsal muscles which were larger than thoracic muscles.After incision of the skin, an 11-gauge Jamshidi needle was placed through the left-side pedicle into the posterior vertebral body. The needle was inserted through the cortex by tapping its back end with a hammer. If the end of the needle reached the inside boundary of the ipsilateral pedicle in the AP view, the lateral view should be checked to see if the end of the needle did not compromise the spinal canal, and safely arrived inside the vertebral body. The entry point of bone was usually made at lateral or supero-lateral wall of the pedicle and there was no artery or nerve (Fig. 4A, B).

Special care was taken to achieve a medial trajectory of the needle and a final midline position of the needle tip in the vertebral body (Fig. 5A, B).

The inflatable bone tamp (IBT) was then positioned within the vertebral body and expanded using direct fluoroscopy and manometric parameters. Inflation continued until vertebral body height was restored, the inflatable bone tamp contacted a vertebral body cortical wall, the IBT reached 250 psi, or the maximal balloon volume was reached. PMMA was prepared with additional barium sulfate. When satisfactory consistency was achieved, PMMA was

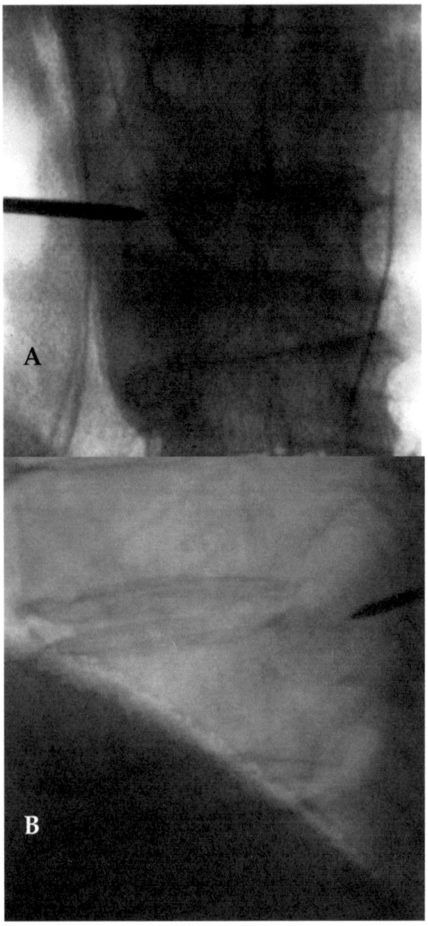

Fig. 4. A-B. Radiographs shows fluoroscopic images at the bone enty point. The needle is anchored at the superolateral area of the pedicle. An anteroposterior view (A) and a lateral view (B).

injected using a commercially available cement delivery system kit under direct fluoroscopic visualization into the cavity in the vertebral body created by an inflatable bone tamp. Cement was administered which produced an excellent filling of the vertebral body cavity (Fig. 6A, B).

The amount of cement injected in the vertebral body is extremely variable—between 3 and 6 mL depending on the metamer, to treat (thoracic or lumbar) and the degree of the collapsed vertebra.

The injection needs to be suspended or terminated if venous, disk space, or epidural extravasation isencountered. Post-procedural CT evaluation is useful to assess correct vertebral PMMA injection and to evaluate complications.All instrumentation removed at the end of the procedure. After the procedure, the patient remains in strict bed rest for 2 hours and is discharged from thehospital after regaining the ability to perambulate, normally the same procedural day.

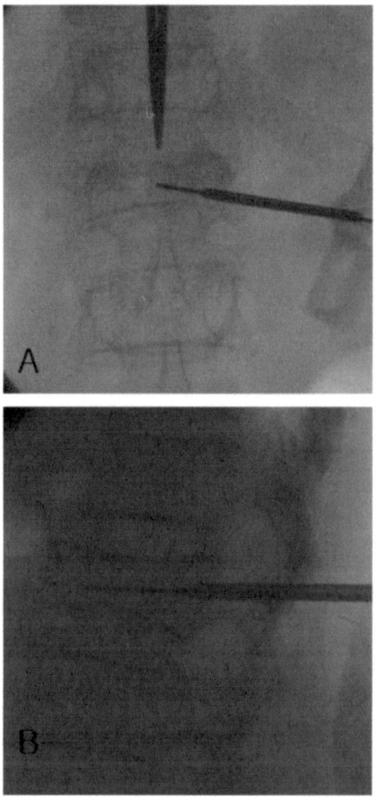

Fig. 5. A-B. Antero-posterior, image of inflatable bone tamp in the midline of the fractured vertebral body.

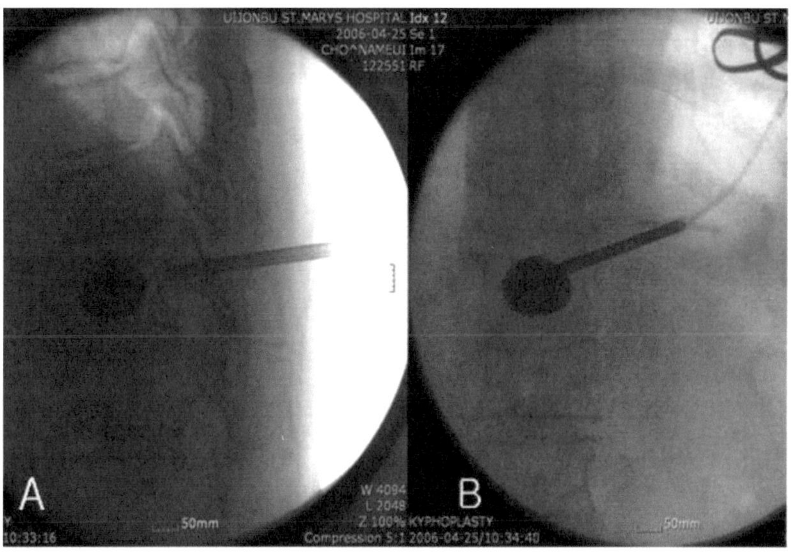

Fig. 6. A) lateral, and B) antero-posterior fluoroscopic image of polymethylmethacrylate filling the cavity within the fractured vertebral body.

5. Postoperative observation and disposal

The vital signs of patients, the cement distribution in the vertebral body and the cement leakage are monitored during the operation. Antibiotics were routinely used within 48 hours. All instrumentation removed at the end of the procedure. After the procedure, the patient remains in strict bed rest for 2 hours and the patients begin to walk on the ground after 6–12 hours. Patients are discharged from the hospital after regaining the ability to perambulate, normally the same procedural day.

6. Technical tip

The key of the single balloon cross-midline expansion with a unipedicular approach is delivering the balloon into the midline position of the vertebral body. A puncturing approach should be made through observing carefully the pedicular route and diameter on the imaging examination before operation. The C-arm was then rotated 10°–20° in an oblique angle ipsilateral with respect to the back being punctured. At this angle, the medial cortex of the pedicle could be visualized clearly. The entry of the needle into the bone should be targeted to a starting point just on the superior and lateral edge of the pedicle projection on the oblique view, so that the maximum transverse angle can be achieved in the pedicular stenotic space without penetrating the media wall of the pedicle. We think the appropriate transverse angle between the needle and the oblique angle of the C-arm was between 3°–5°. This oblique view provided an excellent view of the pedicle during the entire period of needle advancement. Ideally, the IBT should be placed inside the anterior two-thirds of the vertebral body on the lateral view while the tip of the drill overlapped the spinous process of the vertebra under the AP fluoroscopy.

7. Complications

The first step in which it is possible to observe complications is needle and working cannula positioning. The most serious complication is abnormal cement distribution with disk, epidural, or vascular leakage. However, more often leakages are completely asymptomatic. Some types of leakages (intraforaminal, radicular vein) can determine transient radicular pain or thecal sac compression, whereas vascular leakage, in most cases asymptomatic, can lead to symptomatic pulmonary emboli, cerebral infarct, or heart and vascular dissection. This risk is minimized by monitoring the bone filling with a high-quality fluoroscopic unit and by having adequate radiopacity (tantalum) in the cement. Radiculopathy is the major risk with neural foramina leaks (Fig. 7).

Spinal cord compression is an emergency, and urgent surgery is mandatory to prevent neurologic complications. The injection of acrylic cement should be performed under a high-quality fluoroscopic unit. The injection should be immediately interrupted if the cement reaches the posterior cortex of the vertebral body. Adequate radiopacity of acrylic cement (with the addition of tantalum, barium, or tungsten) is mandatory, and the cement should be injected during its pasty polymerization phase.

The filling of an epidural vein and neural foramina cause intercostal neuralgia. Radiculopathy is the major risk with neural foramina leaks. Radiculopathy is particularly difficult to treat at the cervical and lumbar levels. Epidural vein filling does not necessarily cause neuralgia. This complication can be successfully treated with a series of intercostal

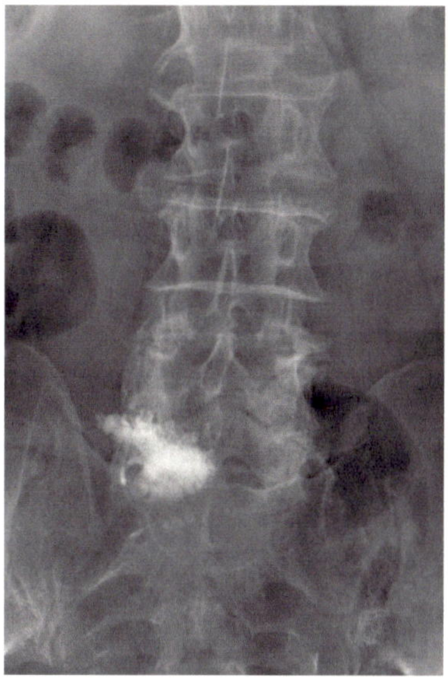

Fig. 7. Antero-posterior X-ray imaging shows leaks toward right neural foramen.

steroid infiltrations. Cement leaks toward the disk usually do not have clinical consequence; however, these leaks may increase the risk of adjacent vertebral collapse.

Leak into paravertebral veins can lead to pulmonary cement embolism (Fig. 8). To avoid major pulmonary infarction, the cement should be injected slowly under fluoroscopic control during its pasty polymerization phase, and the injection should be immediately stopped if a venous leak is observed. Cement leaks into paravertebral soft tissues have no clinical significance.

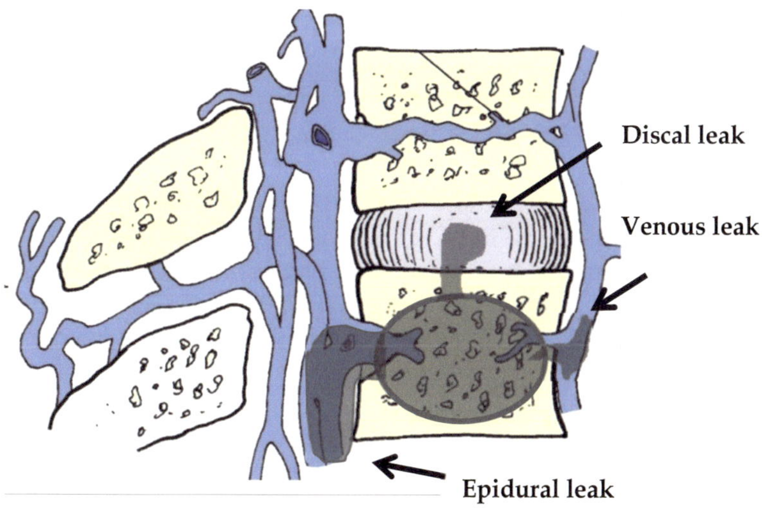

Fig. 8. Drawings show leaks in the sagittal planes.

The second most serious complication is infection. Strict sterility during the intervention is mandatory. Temporary pain can occur after the procedure. Patients are usually free of pain after 24 hours. Post-procedural pain is usually proportional to the volume of cement injected. Most of these patients have good packing of the vertebral body with more than 4 mL of cement injected.

8. Discussion

Percutaneous vertebral augmentation techniques performed with VP or PKP are safe and effective for the treatment of osteoporotic VCF, primary or secondary spine tumors, and selected traumatic fractures. In most cases, VP alone is sufficient to achieve pain relief and quality of life improvement. The advantages of PKP over VP are low-pressure cement injection, the use of high-density cement, and a lower rate of vascular and disk leakage. The disadvantages of KP compared to VP are related to its higher invasiveness, the higher cost (four times higher), the need for deep sedation and time required. The results of the present study indicate that PKP is a minimally invasive procedure aimed at restoring strength, stiffness and is effective in reduction of spinal deformity and in short-term improvement of pain in selected patients with osteoporotic vertebral compression fracture. PKP is a successful technique for pain management and consolidation of pathologic vertebral bodies. The most critical elements for successful PKP are proper patient selection, correct needle placement, good timing of cement injection, strict fluoroscopic control of injection, and operator's experience. The good pain relief obtained with this technique is not correlated with the volume of cement injected, especially in spine metastasis, where 1.5 mL of cement is usually enough to considerably reduce the patient's pain.

The rationale of bilateral transpedicular approach is to achieve adequate endplate elevation with two inflatable bone tamp and to create a large enough cavity for maximal cement filling. With conventional needle trajectories, the inflatable bone tamp remain ipsilateral, thus necessitating bilateral inflatable bone tamp to cover the expanse of the vertebral body.

Previous studies have been suggested that unipedicular kyphoplasty might lead to unilateral wedging or that it would not be as effective in restoring vertebral body height. [1,2,10] Steinmann et al in an ex vivo biomechanical study comparing a bipedicular approach to unipedicuar approach in the treatment of vertebral compression fractures, found no significant lateral wedging associated with unipedicular injections.[10] The unipedicular approach is effective in restoring the vertebral height and vertebral body height was successfully restored by unipedicular kyphoplasty to 96% of fracture levels in our cases. Furthermore, kyphoplasty by unipedicular approach markedly reduced pain and spinal deformity with osteophorotic vertebral compression fracture.A midline-positioned inflatable bone tamp can be inflated to create a large enough cavity in the midline of the vertebral body. Unilateral transpedicular approach has many advantages. This procedure reduced the risk associated with large needle placement. These risks include pedicle fracture, medial transgression of the pedicle or transgression into the spinal canal, nerve injury, cement leakage along the cannula tract, and spinal epidural hematoma.

The key of the single balloon cross-midline expansion with a unipedicular approach is delivering the balloon into the midline position of the vertebral body. First, a puncturing approach should be made through observing carefully the pedicular route and diameter on the imaging examination before operation. Secondly, it was key to try to place the uninflated balloon at the most anterior extent of the vertebral body according to the two fiducial markers denoting the proximal and distal extents of the balloon. Thirdly, those with fractures within two weeks, or back pain exacerbation within two weeks during a longer painful back history, or with a hyper-signal on T2WI in the injured vertebral body on MRI examination, or hypo-signal on both T1WI and T2WI, or with fracture lines and vacuum signs of injured vertebral body on CT scan that predicated old compression fracture and nonunion, i.e. Kümmell's disease are indicated for this technique because the aforementioned are usually signs of fresh fracture or complicated severe osteoporosis. The balloon can be expanded successfully because the resistance of the inflated balloon through liquid pressure was lower.

Even if complications of kyphoplasty are very rare, in previous studies, many authors reported such adverse complication. Coumans et al [7] described a large series of 188 kyphoplasty procedures. There were five cases of complication such as, cement extravasation along the canal. Garfin et al retrospectively reviewed 2194 vertebral compression fractures, finding 3 cases of instrument insertion through the medial pedicle wall, resulting in neurologic injury.[8]

Nussbaum et al [14] also reviewed complications associated with vertebroplasty and kyphoplasty as reported. Kyphoplasty may have an increased risk of pedicle fracture that can lead to spinal compression. It associated with breakage of the pedicle during insertion of the cannula. Theoretically, the incidence of such events may be reduced if unilateral rather than bilateral cannulas are placed. By cannulating only 1 pedicle, one can reasonably assume a considerable reduction in operative time, radiation exposure, and cannulation risks with the unipedicular kyphoplasty when compared to the bipedicular approach. In the procedure that we described, the time required for the procedure was less than 35 minutes and also save the cost about 30% compare to the bipedicular approach.

This procedure has limitation that it is difficult and dangerous to perform the unilateral transpedicular approach in high thoracic level, particularly over the 6th thoracic vertebra, because of small pedicle size and narrow canal. In that case, extrapedicualr approach is more safe and convenient. The surgeon is not satisfied with the inflatable bone tamp position or the extent of inflation or cavity created by using a unipedicular approach, a second contralateral balloon can be placed using the conventional technique. The key to the unilateral approach is the medial trajectory of the needle and the final midline position of the balloon.

9. Conclusion

Balloon kyphoplasty can be performed using a unilateral balloon tamp via a unilateral transpedicular approach for osteoporotic vertebral body compression fracture. There was no greater risk for lateral wedging in the unipedicular group. Given the advantages of a unipedicular approach with respect to vertebral pedicle cannulation risk, operative time, radiation exposure, and cost, this study would support the use of a unilateral transpedicular approach to kyphoplasty in the treatment of osteoporotic vertebral compression fractures.

10. References

[1] Belkoff SM, Mathis JM, Deramond, et al. (2001). An ex vivo biomechanical evaluation of a hydroxyapatite cement for use with kyphoplasty. *Am J Neuroradiol* 22:1212-6.

[2] Belkoff SM, Mathis JM, Fenton DC, et al. (2001). An ex vivo biomechanical evaluation of an inflatable bone tamp used in the treatment of compression fracture. *Spine* 26:151-5.

[3] Berlemann U, Franz T, Orler R, et al. (2004). Kyphoplasty for treatment of osteoporotic vertebral fractures: a prospective non-randomized study. *Eur Spine J* 13:496- 501.

[4] Chiras J. (1997). Percutaneous vertebral surgery: techniques and indications. *J Neuroradiol* 24:45-52.

[5] Cook DJ, Guyatt GH, Adachi JD, et al. (1993). Quality of life issues in women with vertebral fractures due to osteoporosis. *Arthritis Rheum* 36:750-6.

[6] Cotton A, Dewatre F, Cortet B, et al. (1996). Percutaneous vertebroplasty for osteolytic metastases and myeloma: effects of the percentage of lesion filling and the leakage of methyl methacrylate at clinical follow-up. *Radiology* 200:525-30.

[7] Coumans JV, Reinhardt MK, Lieberman IH. (2003). Kyphoplasty for vertebral compression fractures: 1-year clinical outcomes from a prospective study. *J Neurosurg* 99: 44-50.

[8] Garfin S, Lin G, Lieberman I, et al. (2001). Retrospective analysis of the outcomes of balloon kyphoplasty to treat vertebral compression fracture refractory to medical management. *Eur Spine J* 10(suppl 1):S7.

[9] Garfin SR, Yuan HA, Reiley MA. (2001). New technologies in spine: kyphoplasty and vertebroplasty for the treatment of painful osteoporotic compression fractures. *Spine* 26:1511-5.

[10] John Steinmann, DO, Craig T. Tingey, MD, Qian Dai, PhD. (2005). Biomechanical Comparison of Unipedicular Versus Bipedicular Kyphoplasty. *Spine* 30: 201-5.

[11] Kado DM, Browner WS, Palermo L, et al. (1999). Vertebral fractures and mortality in older women. *Arch Intern Med* 159:1215-20.

[12] Lieberman IH, Dudeney S, Reinhardt MK, et al. (2001). Initial outcome and efficacy of kyphoplasty in the treatment of painful osteoporotic vertebral compression fractures. *Spine* 26: 1631-8.

[13] Lyles KW, Gold DT, Shipp KM, et al. (1993). Association of osteoporotic vertebral fractures with impaired functional status. *Am J Med* 94:595-601.

[14] Nussbaum DA, Gailloud P, Murphy K. (2004). A review of complications associated with vertebroplasty and kyphoplasty as reported to the Food and Drug Administration medical device related web site. *J Vasc Interv Radiol* 15:1185-92.

[15] Riggs BL, Melton LJ.(1995). The worldwide problem of osteoporosis: insights afforded by epidemiology. *Bone* 17 (5 Suppl):505S-511S

[16] Rollinghoff M, Sobottke R, Koy T, Delank KS, Eysel P. (2008). Minimally invasive surgery of the lumbar spine. *Z Orthop Unfall* 146:395-408.

[17] Silverman SL. (1992). The clinical consequences of vertebral compression fracture. *Bone* 13(suppl 2):27-31.

2

Osteoporotic Verterbal Compression Fractures

Kook Jin Chung
Department of Orthopaedic Surgery, Kangnam Sacred Heart Hospital,
College of Medicine, Hallym University
Korea

1. Introduction

As the number of old people has been growing, health care of these has been one of major socioeconomic concerns, especially in the developed countries.

Musculoskeletal diseases according to aging process are as much important as medical illness. Based on a report[1], newly diagnosed people with osteoporosis are estimated to affect 200 million women in the world. Because women has lower peak bone mass than men and lose bone mass rapidly right after menopause as they become older. So, osteoporosis imposes a greater burden on women.

The incidence of all osteoporotic vertebral compression fractures increases with age.[2] Shortly after menopause, the incidence of wrist fracture begins to increase and continues to do so until of age of 65, when it plateaus. Vertebral fracture, the most common fracture, occurs earlier after menopause than hip fracture, and continues to rise with age.

Approximately 1.5 million osteoporotic fractures occur in the United States annually, comprised of 250,000 wrist fractures, 250,000 hip fractures, 700,000 vertebral fractures, and 300,000 fractures at other sites. Thus, most common osteoporotic fractures are vertebral fractures. [3-7]

Conventional treatments with bed rest, oral or parenteral analgesics, early ambulation with a brace after relieving symptoms is sufficient to treat osteoporotic vertebral compression factures.

But some patients complain of severe pain that does not respond to these treatments and even show progressive collapse of vertebral bodies and kyphotic deformity with or without neurologic deficits.

Most patients with osteoporotic vertebral compression fractures (OVCFs) well respond to conservative treatments including bed rest, analgesics and immobilization with brace.

But, some of patients complain of uncontrolled persistent chronic pain and progressive collapse of vertebral body, post-traumatic kyphosis with or without neurologic deficits. It is well known that osteoporotic fracture is also associated with significant morbidity and mortality in postmenopausal women.[8-12] There was an approximate 2-fold increase in risk of death following any clinical fracture, primarily due to a 9-fold increase in mortality following vertebral fractures.[13] In contrast, there was no increase in risk of mortality associated with forearm fracture or fractures at sites other than the spine, wrist, or hip.

These data suggest that clinical fractures, particularly vertebral fractures, are associated with an increased risk of mortality in postmenopausal women. Interestingly, the increased mortality following vertebral fracture is comparable to that caused by hip fractures and associated with severe back pain followed by progressive kyphotic deformity and pulmonary dysfunction and its sequelae.

It should be noted that the mechanism behind increased mortality associated with vertebral fractures remains unclear, but may be related more to underlying health status, and co-morbidities rather than the actual fracture itself.[14] Clinical vertebral fractures may be diagnosed more often in women with generally poorer health, a bias that may also contribute to the relationship between vertebral fracture and mortality.

Even though more aggressive treatment may be needed in these complicated cases followed by osteoporotic vertebral compression fractures with majority of patients are not ideal candidates for surgical treatments especially under general anesthesia.

Vertebroplasty was first introduced by Galibert et al in 1987 for the treatment of vertebral body tumor.[15] And then it was adopted as a successful treatment of osteoporotic vertebral compression fractures with advantages of rapid pain relief and long-lasting effect over conventional treatments for several decades. But it has limitation in view of restoration of reduced body heights and leakage of Polymethylmethacrlylate during the procedue.

With the aid of newly designed minimally invasive technique, balloon kyphoplsty the collapsed vertebral body has been reduced satisfactorily by an inflatable bone tamp and then polymethylmethacrylate was safely put into cavity made by bone tamp with less pressure than vertebroplasty. Early results of kyphoplasty for the treatment of osteoporotic vertebral compression fractures has provided restoration of collapsed vertebral body height and reduction of kyphosis, sasitified pain relief and sufficient recovery of daily activity.[16-19]

For those reasons, balloon kyphoplasty has been substituted for vertebroplasty. Thesedays the indication of balloon kyphoplasty has been expanded to include pathological fractures, chronic vertebral fractures and even revision cases. [20-22]

Since the early report described by Garfin et al, bilateral approach using two balloons are usually used to provide en masse reduction for the more efficienct reduction of kyphosis. To the author's knowledge, many surgeons preferred to use bilateral technique. There has been just one study reporting on the clinical result using unilateral kyphoplasty by Boszczyk et al[23] using transcostovertebral approach in mid and high thoracic area. But as well known, osteoporotic verterbral compression fractures usually occurs most commonly in the thoracolumbar junction especially in 12th thoracic and 1st lumbar vertebra. [20,24]

I already reported that the results of comparative study of balloon kyphoplasty with unilateral versus bilateral and unilateral approach in thoracolumbar junction.[25]

Unlike bilateral approach, bone tamp needs to be advanced more to the midline on the anteroposterior view for the purpose of more central placement of balloon in thoracoulumbar junction. (Fig 1,2) According to the result, pain relief was not statistically different but postoperative reduction of fracture and loss of reduction was better in bilateral approach. Although pain score for the two techniques provided same effect, bilateral approach of balloon kyphoplasty can achieve reduction of kyphotic deformity due to an osteoporotic vertebral compression fractures to gain good sagittal alignment. (Fig 3-A,B) fractures occurred in mid and high thoracic spine and cases not requiring so much reduction for restoration of kyphosis.[24,25]

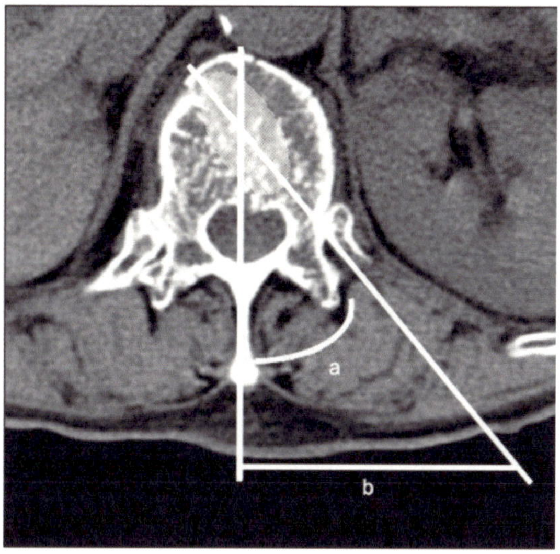

Fig. 1. Balloon kyphoplasty using unilateral Approach. The angle (a) formed by the two lines connecting the most ventral portion of the vertebral body and the spinous process and the line is placing balloon in the middle of the vertebral body, distance (b) between the two points where these two lines contacted the body surface.

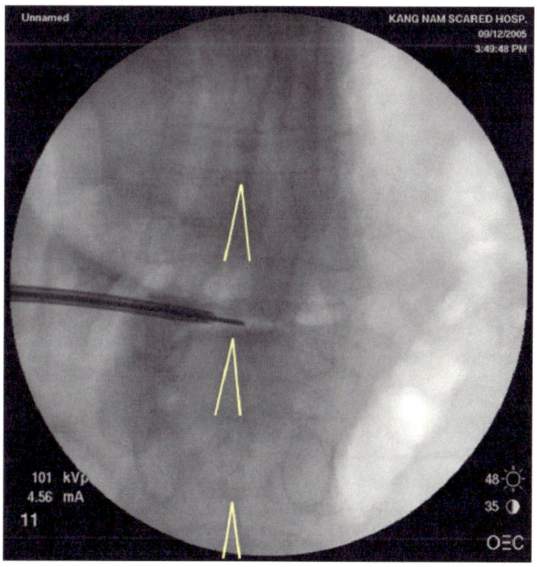

Fig. 2. Bone tamp is advanced to the midline on the anteroposterior view under the C-arm image intensifier.

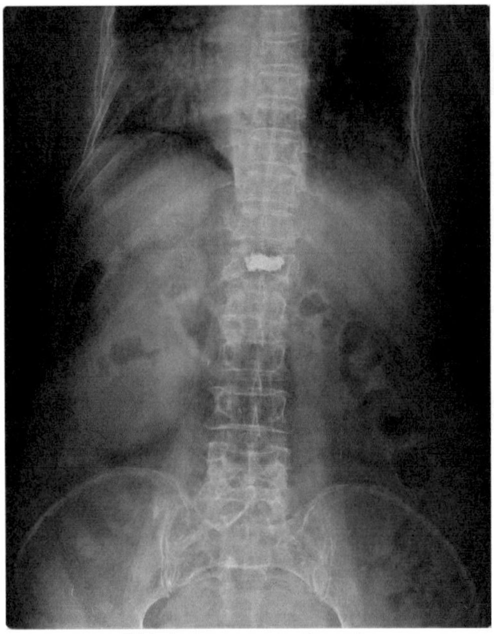

(A) Anteroposterior view

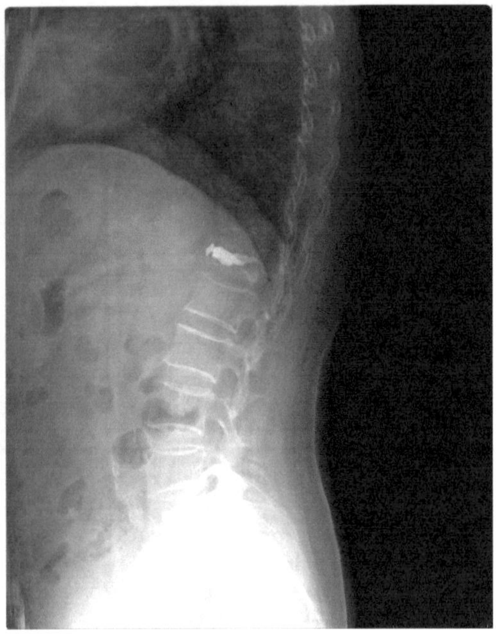

(B) Lateral view

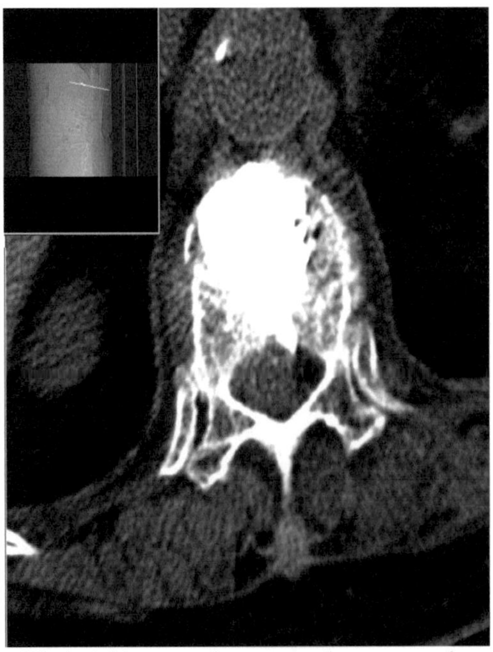

(C) Axial image of computed tomography

Fig. 3. Balloon Kyphoplasty using Unilateral approach

There is no doubt that prevention of osteoporotic vertebral compression fractures is more important than surgical treatment. But in fractures not responding to prevention and conservative treatments, timely surgical intervention can afford to provide good reduction of fracture and correction of kyphosis and recovery of activity of daily living.

2. References

[1] Iqbal MM. Osteoporosis: Epidemilolgy, diagnosis, and treatment. South Med J 2000;93:2-18.

[2] Wasnich RD: Primer on the Metabolic Bone Diseases and Metabolism. 4th edition, 1999

[3] Riggs and Melton, *New Eng J Med* 1986;314:1676-86.

[4] Cooper C, Atkinson EJ, Jacobsen SJ et al. Population-based study of survival after osteoporotic fractures. Am J Epidemiol 1993;137:1001-1005.

[5] Truumees E, Hilibrand A, Vaccaro AR Percutaneous vertebral augmentation Spine J 2004;4:218-229.

[6] Zoarski GH, Snow P, Olan WJ et al. Percutaneous vertebroplasty for osteporotic compression fractures: Quantitiative prospective evaluation of long-term outcomes J Vasc Interv Radiol 2002;13:139-148.

[7] Riggs BL, Melton LJ III The worldwide problem of osteoporosis : Insights afforded by epidemiology Bone 1995;17:505S-511S.

[8] Cooper C, Atkinson EJ, O'Fallon WM et al Incidence of clinically diagnosed vertebral fractures: A population based study in Rochester, MN, 1985-1989 J Bone Miner Res 1992;7:221-227.

[9] Coumans JV, Reinhardt MK, Lieberman IH Kyphoplasty for vertebral compression fractures: 1-year clinical outcomes froma prospective study. J Neurosurg 2003;99:44-50.

[10] Lyles KW, Gold DT, Shipp KM et al Association of osteoporotic vertebral compression fractures with impaired functional status Am J Med 1993;94:595-601.

[11] Evans AJ, Jensen ME, Kip KE et al Vertebral compression fractures: Pain reduction and improvement in functional mobility after percutaneous polymethylmethacrylate vertebroplasty retrospective report of 245 cases Radiology 2003;226:366-372.

[12] Kado DM, Duong T, Stone KL et al Incident vertebral fractures and mortality on older women: A prospective study Osteoporosis IOnt 2003;14:589-594.

[13] Cauley JA et al., *Osteoporos Int* 2000;11:556-561.

[14] Browner WS et al., *Arch Int Med* 1996;156:1521-1525.

[15] Galibert P, Deramond H. Note préliminaire sur le traitement sed angiomes vertébraux par vertébroplastie acrylique percutanée. Neurochirurgie 1987;33:166-167.

[16] Eck JC, Hodges SD, Humphreys SC Vertebroplasty: A new treatment strategy for osteoporotic compression fractures. Am J Orthop 2002;31:123-128.

[17] Watts NB, Harris ST, Genant HK Treatment of painful osteoporotic vertebral fractures with percutaneous vertebroplasty or kyphoplasty Osteoporosis Int 2001;12:429-437.

[18] Garfin SR, Yuan HA, Reiley MA new technologies in spine: Kyphoplasty and vertebroplasty for the treatment of painful osteoporotic compression fractures. Spine 2001;26:1511-1515.

[19] Lieberman IH, Dudeney S, Reinhardt MK, Bell G Initial outcome and efficacy of kyphoplasty in the treatment of painful osteoporotic vertebral compression fractures. Spine 2001;26:1631-1638.

[20] Ledlie J, Renfro M Balloon kyphoplasty: one-year outcomes in vertebral body height restoration, chronic pain and activity levels J Neurosurg 2003;26:1631-1638.

[21] Gaitanis IN, Hadjipavlou AG, Katonis PG, Tzermiadianosi MN, Pasku DS, Patwardhan AG Balloon kyphoplasty for the treatment of pathological vertebral compressive fractures. Eur Spine J 2005;14:250-260.

[22] Yoon ST, Quershi AA, Heller JG, Nordt JC 3rd Kyphoplasty for salvage of a failed vertebroplasty in osteoporotic vertebral compression fractures : case report and surgical technique. J Spinal Disord Tech;18(Suppl):S129-134.

[23] Boszczyk B, Bierschneider M, Hauck S, Beisse R, Potulski M, Jacsche H Transcostovertebral kyphoplasty of the mid and high thoracicspine Eur Spine J 2005;14:992-999.

[24] Lee YL, Yip KM The osteoporotic spine Clin Orthop Relat Res 1999;323:91-97.

[25] Chung HJ, Chung KJ, Yoon HS, Kwon IH Comparative study of blloon kyphoplasty with unilateral versus bilateral approach in osteoporotic vertebral compression fractures Int Orthop 2008;32:817-820.

3

Nonunion of Osteoporotic Vertebral Fractures: Clinical Characteristics and Surgical Treatment

Genlin Wang and Huilin Yang*
Department of Orthopaedics, The First Affiliated Hospital of Soochow University, Suzhou, Jiangsu Province, China

1. Introduction

Osteoporotic vertebral fractures (OVFs) are a frequently encountered clinical problem with an estimated incidence of 700,000 per year in the United States. Additionally, they are becoming more common as the median age of the population continues to increase.[1-2] OVFs may be a sentinel sign of failing health in elderly patients. The degree of kyphosis correlates well with the patient's physical function, the risk of further fractures, compression of the spinal cord, and pulmonary function.[3-5] Any of these factors may contribute to an increased mortality.[4, 6-7] Patients with OVFs, who are refractory to conservative treatments, have been operated on by vertebroplasty or kyphoplasty over the past years.[8-16] The fracture nonunion of OVF's has recently become an interesting topic of focus. This nonunion is often unrecognized and left untreated. This is unfortunate since, unlike acute vertebral compression fractures (VCFs), nonunion does not heal with time and will be a continued source of chronic pain and disability for the patient.[17] The aim of this article is to review the etiology of the fracture nonunion, clinical situation, imaging characteristics, and surgical treatment of the nonunion. Vertebroplasty and kyphoplasty, two recently developed operative procedures, will be reviewed and discussed in the management of OVFs.

2. Etiology

The etiology of the nonunion of OVFs is not very clear as there are many factors that can cause the nonunion. Some scholars[18-19] believed that osteoporotic patients had a lower ability of osteogenesis in addition to their age-related microarchitectural deterioration of vertebrae which would subsequently lead to the nonunion or delayed union. There is evidence of this hypothesis from animal models. Namkung-Matthail et al [20] showed a 40% reduction of callus formation in the cross-sectional area and a 23% reduction in bone mineral density in the healing femur of an osteoporotic rat model. There are several possible explanations for this effect. Bergman et al [21] reported that there might be fewer mesenchymal stem cells (MSCs) in osteoporotic mice. They also stated that defects in the number and proliferative potential of MSCs might underlie age-related defects in osteoblast number and function. This may explain the age-related decrease in the number of osteoblasts.[18] Rodriguez et al[19] also reported mesenchymal stem cells in post-menopausal women differed from those in the premenopausal

* Corresponding Author

by having a lower rate of growth as well as a deficiency in their ability to differentiate along the osteogenic lineage. Thus, vertebral fractures in elderly patients with severe osteoporosis may experience nonunion. This indicates that the ability to form bone is reduced in elderly patients with severe osteoporosis or deteriorated bone metabolism.

The nonunion of OVFs is thought to be related to avascular necrosis of the vertebral body and has been referred to as Kummel's disease of the spine.[22-23] Ratcliffe[24] has verified vascular supply in the anterior region beneath the superior endplate is the most tenuous by microarteriography. OVFs often occur in the anterior vertebrae where blood supply is easily destroyed which can lead to nonunion. This may explain why intraosseous clefts occurred primarily in the anterosuperior portion of the vertebral body.[14, 17] Baba et al [25] believed that fibrous granulation tissue and necrotic bone in collapsed vertebral bodies changed vascular supply in the injured region and influenced the fracture union. This fibrous granulation tissue and necrotic bone result in the formation of pseudarthroses. [26] A vascular insult can cause ischemic necrosis of the vertebral body and form the intraosseous clefts, [22, 27] leading to delayed union or nonunion[28]. Recent studies have shown that these clefts are frequent and represent fracture nonunion in patients with OVFs.[29-31]

However, Kim et al [32] reported 67 vacuum phenomena among 652 osteoporotic VCFs and discussed that biomechanics, not ischemic or avascular theory, may play an important role in this phenomenon. Yuan et al [33] biomechanically demonstrated the thoracolumbar junction is the spinal region which receives the greatest dynamic load, and therefore may predispose to fracture nonunion.

Infections, steroids, radiotherapy, angiitis, pancreatitis, cirrhosis, alcoholism, atherosclerosis, old age and osteoporosis are considered to be high risk factors of OVFs to progress to nonunion. We find old age and osteoporosis are major risk factors, this may be related to our case-selection. [34]

3. Clinical situation

There is no epidemiological data about incidence and age of onset. The nonunion of OVFs mainly occurs at the thoracolumbar junction.[14, 17, 32] Most of the patients have no nerve lesion. The cardinal symptom is back pain with a certain feature that is distinctly proportional to activity and position. The pain is almost completely relieved by rest, most often in a lateral decubitus position, while symptoms return as soon as the spine is loaded in an attempt to sit, stand, or walk.[16-17] These patients' pattern of pain is highly suggestive of this diagnosis. The back pain may be attributed to pseudarthrosis or to spinal deformity such as kyphosis or kyphoscoliosis which can produce a kaleidoscope of problems.[35] However, motion of this intravertebral dynamic mobility is the primary cause of severe back pain.[14, 16, 36] Toyone et al [37] examined 100 consecutive patients with OVFs, and analyzed changes in vertebral wedging rate between the supine and standing position, and its association with back pain. There was a significant correlation between the changes in vertebral wedging rate and back pain and between the supine and standing position and back pain. This finding gives insight into the pathogenesis of the back pain.

4. Imaging features

The nonunion of OVFs may show intravertebral clefts [31] or so-called vacuum phenomena [17, 22, 32] on vertebral imaging views most of which locate in the anterior region of vertebral body.[14, 17] These clefts indicating fracture nonunion can easily be missed on standing lateral radiographs.[29-31] However, they can be accentuated on lateral view radiographs with hyperextension.[17, 22, 32]

Peh et al[38] reported vacuum phenomena in only 9% of patients in a retrospective study of lateral radiographs thus reflecting the poor sensitivity of lateral radiographs in detecting the clefts. McKiernan et al [14] reported 50 consecutive patients with 82 OVFs in a prospective radiographic study and stated that clefts were detectable by standing lateral radiography in 14% of the cases, by supine cross-table radiography in 64%, and MRI in 96%. A cleft can be detected on T2-weighted MRI as an area of high or low signal intensity depending on whether it contains fluid or gas and on the repositioning of the patient's spine with time.[39, 40] However, recent studies[13, 17] have reported that clefts of the fracture nonunion show high signal intensity on T2-weighted MRI. The clearly defined hyperintense intraosseous signal observed on T2-weighted sagittal MR[13, 17, 41] may yet be a proven pathognomonic of this diagnosis. However, MRI may lead to false positives. Lane et al [31], in a retrospective analysis, reported intravertebral clefts in 31.8% of patients during percutaneous vertebroplasty, 52.8% of which had been detected on pre-operative MRI.

No cleft can be observed on a fresh-fractured vertebrae.[37] Only in the absence of fracture union and with persistent mobility may clefts appear with their margins becoming increasingly sclerotic with time.[14, 17, 37] Dynamic mobility, a recently recognized property of some osteoporotic vertebral compression fractures, may also appear. Dynamic mobility, [42] a change of vertebral height or configuration with changes in body positioning, is demonstrated by stress views in x-rays.[14, 41] It can be determined when anterior vertebral height varies when comparing standing with supine lateral radiographs.[14] The characteristics and significance of dynamic mobility are not well investigated. The OVFs is usually associated with intravertebral clefts and greater fracture severity.[14, 17, 29-30, 43] Yoon et al[17] believed motion of the endplates at the level of the fracture and an intraosseous vacuum sign represented a persistent, mobile nonunion. Jang et al[41] also thought the changes in the anterior vertebral height on the dynamic lateral flexion and extension views confirmed intravertebral fracture nonunion.

Flexion/extension or standing/supine lateral radiographs reveal that mobile fractures are capable of postural correction by extension of the spine[35]. Substantial correction of kyphosis and anterior vertebral height can be corrected by extended posture. Kyphoplasty or vertebroplasty in addition to this extended posture can also correct the spinal instability that results from the mobile vertebral body.[41] The restoration of vertebral body height might not only be position dependent, but time dependent as well. McKiernan et al[14] had 14 patients with OVFs confined to the supine position overnight. These patients had additional vertebral height restoration. He termed this delayed postural vertebral fracture reduction "latent mobility." Dynamic mobility and latent mobility are undoubtedly manifestations of the same process of fracture nonunion. The importance of postural reduction should not be underestimated. The mobility can contribute significantly to vertebral height restoration. Using the technique of postural reduction may result in sufficient vertebral height restoration to allow vertebroplasty to be safely performed in some patients in whom the procedure had otherwise been deemed technically impossible or unsafe.[14-15]

5. Treatment

Most OVFs are managed with a short period of rest or activity modification, narcotic analgesics, and a brace.[44] However, patients with fracture nonunion that are refractory to conservative treatments continue to have persistent back pain, progressive vertebral body collapse and kyphosis, and mobility of the fracture.[17] These patients often need vertebroplasty or kyphoplasty intervention to make back pain disappear.[12, 30-32] However, there is not a consensus on whether to select vertebroplasty or kyphoplasty.

Some scholars[15, 45, 46] have that believed percutaneous vertebroplasty is effective for treating the fracture nonunion. Ha et al[45] found the difference between patients with and without a cleft in the Oswertry Disability Index (ODI) and visual analog scale (VAS) scores at the final follow-up was not statistically significant. This agrees with the results of McKiernan et al. [29] Krauss et al [46] also found pain reduction to be the same in both groups, but patients with intravertebral clefts showed a significant reduction of the kyphosis angle compared to non-cleft patients during vertebroplasty.

Injecting cement into part of an intraosseous cleft will allow even cement filling of the entire cleft. Chen et al[15] believed that a compression fracture with a vacuum cleft could be treated successfully with a uni-pedicle approach. Enlargement of the cleft by postural reduction can restore the vertebral body height in mobile fractured vertebrae with nonunion. Thus, Krauss et al[46] believed that kyphoplasty is not necessary for the nonunion. However, Garfin et al[9] and Yoon et al[17] thought kyphoplasty offers the additional advantages of restoring vertebral body height and correcting kyphosis with the use of sufficient cement volume. Conversely, they believed that vertebroplasty probably led to inadequate initial fixation of a mobile nonunion which would result in clinical failure. Grohs et al[16] carried an open prospective investigation of the efficacy of balloon kyphoplasty in the treatment of intravertebral pseudarthrosis. This study found that the extent of reduction of kyphosis and the duration of pain relief differed in regards to the type of fracture. In case of moderate to severe kyphosis occurring at thoracolumbar junction followed by nonunion of osteoporotic vertebral fractures, the results of verterboplasty or kyphoplasty treatment in view of reduction of kyphosis and loss of kyphosis are limited. To enable a better comparison of kyphosis reduction by vertebroplasty and kyphoplasty, a prospective study comparing both procedures should be performed.

Although percutaneous vertebroplasty and percutaneous kyphopalsty offer an efficient and safe treatment option, they are not free of complications. The main complication is polymethyl methacrylate (PMMA) leakage. Reported PMMA leakage rates vary. By CT scan after vertebroplasty, Jung et al[13] found that the leakage rate was 55.5% in patients with clefts and 51.0% in patients without clefts (i.e. no significant difference). Ha et al[45] compared the results of vertebroplasty in OVFs with and without clefts. More leakage occurred in the presence of a cleft with an incidence of 86.7%. These findings were consistent with those of Yeom et al [47-48]. This higher rate, compared to that of compression fractures without intravertebral vacuum clefts, may be attributed to the presence of a cleft. However, Krauss et al[46] compared the occurrence of cement leaks after vertebroplasty. Cement leakage occurred in 18.2% of cases with clefts and in 46% of regular osteoporotic fractures without clefts. Patients with intravertebral clefts have a significantly lower risk of experiencing cement leakage during vertebroplasty and usually require a smaller amount of cement per vertebra. The reason might be that an intravertebral cleft is an avascular process surrounded by a fibrocartilaginous membrane.

Cement leakage types differed in osteoporotic compression fractures with and without intravertebral vacuum clefts. Jung et al[13] reported that the leakage types were intradiscal (65.0%), perivertebral venous (25%), epidural (5%), and foraminal (5%) in compression fractures with clefts; and epidural (44.0%), perivertebral venous (32%), and intradiscal (24%) in those without clefts. A significant difference was found between the most frequent types in both groups (P = 0.006, P = 0.003, respectively). Intradiscal type was 65%, lower than the 79% reported by Peh et al.[38]. Krauss et al[46] found that there was one cement leakage into a paravertebral vein in the cleft group while other leakage was through fractured endplates into the intervertebral discs. Higher leakage of the intradiscal type may be associated with intravertebral clefts. This suggestion is based on the findings that leakage into the disc almost always occurred at the location of the cleft as reported in the series of Peh et al. [38] It is important to note that the risk of cement leakage is generally less in kyphoplasty than for percutaneous vertebroplasty because the bone cement is injected under lower pressure and can be more viscous when injected.[16, 17, 49] We also found the advantages of kypjoplasty over vertebroplasty are lower incidence of PMMA leakage and better correction of kyphotic deformity for nonunion of OVFs.[50]

6. Conclusion

OVFs, like other fractures, may develop nonunion which can often go unrecognized. There are many factors that cause the nonunion such as lower ability of osteogenesis and age-related microarchitectural deterioration of vertebrae and avascular necrosis of the vertebral body. Also, biomechanics may predispose to fracture nonunion. The nonunion of OVFs may show intravertebral clefts on vertebral imaging views. These intravertebral clefts most often locate in the anterior region of the vertebral body. Flexion/extension or standing/supine lateral radiographs can reveal fracture mobility. The importance of postural reduction should not be underestimated. Substantial correction of kyphosis and the anterior vertebral height may be obtained by an extended posture for spinal instability caused by mobility of the vertebral body. The cardinal symptom is back pain which is refractory to conservative treatments. These patients often need operative intervention. At present, the best surgical treatment option may be vertebroplasty and kyphoplasty. However, the long-term outcome of cement injection into the vertebral body is unclear. It is possible that injected cement may increase the stresses at adjacent levels and thus increase the likelihood of fractures at those levels. Development of bone cements with good long-term biocompatibility and mechanical properties that are similar to vertebrae may be a better and more viable solution.

7. References

[1] Riggs BL, Melton LJ 3rd. Involutional osteoporosis. N Engl J Med, 1986, 314: 1676-1686.

[2] Rao RD, Singrakhia MD. Painful osteoporotic vertebral fracture: pathogenesis, evaluation, and roles of vertebroplasty and kyphoplasty in its management. J Bone Joint Sug (Am) 2003, 85-A(10):2010-2022.

[3] Pluijm SM, Tromp AM, Smit JH, Deeg DJ, Lips P. Consequences of vertebral deformities in older men and women. J Bone Miner Res 2000;15:1564-72.

[4] Kado DM, Browner WS, Palermo L, et al. Vertebral body fractures and mortality in older women: a prospective study. Arch Intern Med 1999;159:1215-20.

[5] Yang HL, Zhao LJ, Liu JY, et al. Changes of Pulmonary Function for Patients With Osteoporotic Vertebral Compression Fractures After Kyphoplasty. J Spinal Disord Tech, 2007, 20: 221-225.

[6] Linville DA 2nd. Vertebroplasty and kyphoplasty. South Med J 2002;95:583-7.

[7] Cotten A, Boutry N, Cortet B, et al. Percutaneous vertebroplasty: state of the art. Radiographics, 1998; 18:311-20.

[8] Cortet B, Cotton A, Boutry N, et al. Percutaneous vertebroplasty in the treatment of osteoporotic vertebral compression fractures. *J Rheumatol* 1999;26:2222-8.

[9] Garfin SR, Yuan HA, Reiley MA. New technologies in spine: kyphoplasty and vertebroplasty for the treatment of painful osteoporotic compression fractures. *Spine.* 2001;26:1511-1515.

[10] Peters K, Guiot B, Martin P, et al. Vertebroplasty for osteoporotic compression fractures: current practice and evolving techniques. *Neurosurgery* 2002;51:96–103.

[11] Berlemann U, Franz T, Orler R, et al. Kyphoplasty for treatment of osteoporotic vertebral fractures: a prospective non-randomized study. *Eur Spine J* 2004;13:496–501.

[12] Carlier RY, Gordji H, Mompoint DM, et al. Osteoporotic vertebral collapse: percutaneous vertebroplasty and local kyphosis correction. Radiology. 2004;233:891-898.

[13] Jung JY, Lee MH, Ahn JM. Leakage of polymethylmethacrylate in percutaneous vertebroplasty: comparison of osteoporotic vertebral compression fractures with and without an intravertebral vacuum cleft. J Comput Assist Tomogr, 2006, 30: 501-506.

[14] McKiernan F, Faciszewski T. Intravertebral clefts in osteoporotic vertebral compression fractures. Arthritis Rheum, 2003, 48: 1414-1419.

[15] Chen LH, Lai PL, Chen WJ. Unipedicle percutaneous vertebroplasty for spinal intraosseous vacuum cleft. Clin Orthop, 2005, 435: 148-153.

[16] Grohs JG., Matzner M, Trieb K, et al. Treatment of intravertebral pseudarthroses by balloon Kyphoplasty. J Spinal Disord Tech, 2006, 19: 560-565.

[17] Yoon ST, Qureshi AA, Heller JG, et al. Kyphoplasty for salvage of a failed vertebroplasty in osteoporotic vertebral compression fractures: case report and surgical technique. J Spinal Disord Tech, 2005, 18: S129-S134.

[18] D'Ippolito G, Schiller PC, Ricordi C, et al. Age-related osteogenic potential of mesenchymal stromal stem cells from human vertebral bone marrow. J Bone Miner Res, 1999, 14: 1115-1122.

[19] Rodriguez JP, Garat S, Gajardo H, et al. Abnormal osteoporotic patients is reflected by altered mesenchymal stem cells dynamics. *J Cell Biochem*, 1999, 75: 414-23.

[20] Namkung-Matthail H, Appleyard R, Jansen J, et al. Osteoporosis influences the early period of fracture healing in a rat osteoporotic model. Bone 2001;28:80-6.

[21] Bergman RJ, Gazit D, Kahn AJ, et al. Age-related changes in osteogenic stem cells in mice. J Bone Miner Res 1996;11:568-77.

[22] Maldaque BE, Noel HM, Malghem JJ. The intravertebral vacuum cleft: a sign of ischemic vertebral collapse. Radiology. 1978;129:23-29.

[23] Assmann H, Montag M, Krzok G, Endert G. Related articles, links [Case reports of the Kummel-Verneuil syndrome] (German). *Rev Med Chir Soc Med Nat Iasi.* 1992;96:103-106.
[24] Ratcliffe JF. The arterial anatomy of the adult human lumbar vertebral body. J Anat 1980;131:57–79.
[25] Baba H, Maezawa Y, Kamitani K, et al. Osteoporotic vertebral collapse with late neurological complications. Paraplegia, 1995, 33(5):281-289.
[26] Hasegawa K, Homma T, Uchiyama S. Vertebral pseudoarthrosis in the osteoporotic spine. Spine. 1998;23:2201–2206.
[27] Bhalla S, Reinus WR: The linear intravertebral vacuum: A sign of benign vertebral collapse. AJR Am J Roentgenol 170:1563-1569, 1998.
[28] Ito Y, Hasegawa Y, Toda K, et al. Pathogenesis and diagnosis of delayed vertebral collapse resulting from osteoporotic spinal fracture. Spine J. 2002;2:101-106.
[29] McKiernan F, Jensen R, Faciszewski T. The dynamic mobility of vertebral compression fractures. J Bone Miner Res. 2003;18:24-29.
[30] Mirovsky Y, Anekstein Y, Shalmon E, et al. Vacuum clefts of the vertebral bodies. AJNR Am J Neuroradiol. 2005;26:1634-1640.
[31] Lane JI, Maus TP, Wald JT, et al. Intravertebral clefts opacified during vertebroplasty: pathogenesis, technical implications, and prognostic significance. AJNR Am J Neuroradiol. 2002;23:1642-1646.
[32] Kim DY, Lee SH, Jang JS, et al. Intravertebral vacuum phenomenon in osteoporotic compression fracture: report of 67 cases with quantitative evaluation of intravertebral instability. J Neurosurg. 2004;100:24-31.
[33] Yuan HA, Brown CW, Phillips FM. Osteoporotic spinal deformity: a biomechanical rationale for the clinical consequence and treatment of vertebral body compression fractures. J Spinal Disord Tech, 2004;17: 236-242.
[34] Wang G, Yang H, Jiang WM, et al. Balloon kyphoplasty for osteoporotic vertebral compression fractures with osteonecrosis. Chin J surg, 2010, 48: 593-596.
[35] Hadjipavlou AG, Tzermiadianos MN, Katonis PG, Szpalski M. Percutaneous vertebroplasty and balloon kyphoplasty for the treatment of osteoporotic vertebral compression fractures and osteolytic tumours. J Bone J Jiont Surg (Br), 2005, 87: 1595-1604.
[36] Laloux P, Lefebvre S, Esselinckx W. Spinal cord compression secondary to vertebral aseptic osteonecrosis. Spine. 1991;16: 480-481.
[37] Toyone T, Tanaka T, Wada Y, et al. Changes in vertebral wedging rate between supine and standing position and its association with back pain: a prospective study in patients with osteoporotic vertebral compression fractures. Spine, 2006, 31: 2963-2966.
[38] Peh WC, Gelbart MS, Gilula LA, Peck DD. Percutaneous vertebroplasty: treatment of painful vertebral compression fractures with intraosseous vacuum phenomena. *AJR Am J Roentgenol* 2003;180:1411-17.
[39] Malghem J, Maldague B, Labaisse MA, et al. Intravertebral vacuum cleft: changes in content after supine positioning. *Radiology.* 1993;187:483-487.
[40] Naul LG, Peet GJ, Maupin WB. Avascular necrosis of the vertebral body: MR imaging. *Radiology.* 1989;172:219-222.

[41] Jang JS, Kim DY, Lee SH. Efficacy of Percutaneous Vertebroplasty in the Treatment of Intravertebral Pseudarthrosis Associated With Noninfected Avascular Necrosis of the Vertebral Body, Spine, 2003, 28: 1588-1592.

[42] Faciszewski T, McKiernan F. Calling all vertebral fractures: a consensus for comparison of treatment and outcome. J Bone Miner Res 2002; 17:185–191.

[43] McKiernan F, Faciszewski T. The modal distribution of osteoporotic vertebral compression fracture types. J Bone Miner Res 2002; 17(suppl):S260–S261.

[44] Kallmes DF, Jensen ME. Percutaneous vertebroplasty. Radiology 2003; 229:27–36.

[45] Ha KY, Lee JS, Kim KW, Chon JS. Percutaneous vertebroplasty for vertebral compression fractures with and without intravertebral clefts.J Bone Joint Surg (Br): 2006, 88: 629-633.

[46] Krauss M, Hirschfelder H, Tomandl B, Lichti G, Bär I. Kyphosis reduction and the rate of cement leaks after vertebroplasty of intravertebral clefts. Eur Radiol, 2006 16: 1015–1021.

[47] Yeom JS, Kim WJ, Choy WS, et al. Bone cement leakage in vertebroplasty for osteoporotic compression fractures. J Kor Ortho Asso 2003;38:293-300.

[48] Yeom JS, Kim WJ, Choy WS, et al. Leakage in cement in percutaneous transpedicular vertebroplasty for painful osteoporotic compression fractures. J Bone Joint Surg [Br] 2003;85-B:83-9.

[49] Lieberman IH, Dudeney S, Reinhardt M-K, et al. Initial outcomes and efficacy of "kyphoplasty" in the treatment of painful osteoporotic vertebral compression fractures. Spine. 2001; 26:1631-1638.

[50] Wang G, Yang H, Chen K. Osteoporotic vertebral compression fractures with an intravertebral cleft treated by percutaneous balloon kyphoplasty. J Bone Joint Surg-Br. 2010; 92: 1553-1557.

4

The Research on Bolster for Self-Replacement Combined with Percutaneous Vertebroplasty in Treatment of Vertebral Compression Fractures

Mo Wen[1], Cheng Shaodan[2] and Hu Zhijun[1]

[1]*Department of Orthopedics,Longhua Hospital, Shanghai University of Traditional Chinese Medicine, Shanghai*

[2]*Department of Lu' s Traumatology,Huashan Hospital,Fudan University, Jing'an Branch, Shanghai, China*

1. Introduction

Percutaneous vertebroplasty (PVP) is a minimally invasive spinal surgery technique arising in the past 20 years, which has been widely used in the treatment of vertebral compression fractures (VCF). However, people have gradually found that the approach can not completely restore the vertebral height and has a high incidence of leakage, etc. From August 2006 to August 2007, 26 cases of VCF underwent traditional bolster for self-replacement treatments before PVP; furthermore, we conducted from 1 to 12 months of follow-up visits. The results are as follows.

2. Materials and methods

2.1 Clinical materials

There were 6 men and 20 women in the 26 cases of VCF studied. Ages ranged from 51 to 80 years, with a mean of 64.5 years. There was one case in the 51 to 55 age range, 4 cases in the 56 to 60 age range, 14 cases in the 61 to 70 age range and 7 cases in the 71 to 80 age range; 5 cases involved a single thoracic body, 6 cases involved 1 thoracic body and 1 lumbar body, 8 cases involved a single lumbar body, 6 cases involved 2 lumbar bodies and 1 case involved 3 lumbar bodies; all cases were osteoporotic vertebral compression fractures, duration of 1 to 15 days. At admission to hospital and before surgery patients had no neurological symptoms or signs of root damage. Preoperative CT scans of vertebra showed a complete posterior vertebral body.

2.2 Therapeutic methods

2.2.1 Bolster for self-replacement: When patients were admitted to hospital,they were laid on a hard bed with a bolster under the waist. This could be tolerated in the case of daily elevation of the pillow (generally a maximum of 10cm), so that the spine was hyper extended, for 3 to 7 days; in the meantime, patients were encouraged to adopt the "five-point support method" exercise as soon as possible, to aid reset.

2.2.2 PVP treatment: General admission electrocardiogram and other tests were used to understand the patient's conditions as well as the function of important organs .Blood glucose , prothrombin time,liver and kidney function tests as well as iodine allergy tests were completed to exclude the possibility of surgical contraindications.

A preparation of 0.09g luminal was taken orally for preoperative sedation. Surgery was performed with patients in the prone position,the two shoulders and two iliacs were elevated; puncturing and injecting of bone cement was achieved using a pressurized syringe device (Israel Disc-0-Tech). The bone cement was a special bone cement used for the PVP / PKP (polymethylmethacrylate, PMMA, Tianjin Synthetic Material Research Institute products).

The operation was carried out under the surveillance of the C-arm, all adaptors were used with a unilateral needle (vertebral compression heavier side in the anteroposterior position). Thoracic and lumbar punctures were achieved through the lateral vertebral neck. An anteroposterior fluoroscopy C-arm tube was used to adjust the angle so that both lateral vertebral necks showed clearly,two Kirschner wires crossed and were fixed on the skin surface, the surface projection of lateral vertebral neck coincided with the intersection of the two Kirschner wires.The puncture point lay slightly outside and above,1 ~ 1.5cm from the coincidence point. After local anesthesia, keeping the transfixion pin and sagittal body appearing 15 ° ~ 30 ° angle,after the transfixion pin got into the lateral vertebral neck, then pushed the transfixion pin 1 ~ 2cm. Checking under lateral fluoroscopy to confirm correct transfixion point,Penetrated with slow rotation, so that the transfixion pin tip was in the central of vertebral body in the anteroposterior and the anterior 1 / 3 in the lateral;Then injected 3~ 5 mL of iohexol contrast agent, observed the contrast agent to confirm the filling of the vertebral body. If there was no significant vascular leakage, then connected the rotation pressure syringe, slowly pushed the cement into the vertebral body under fluoroscopy.

When bone cement was near the posterior margin of the vertebral body,stopped pushing.

If injection caused local gas pains, pains in the legs, numbness or burning feeling ,stopped injecting for a moment. If the sensory disturbances disappeared within 30s ,the patients had good locomotor activity, bone cement did not exceed the posterior margin of the vertebral body for 3mm,we could continue to inject.

After injection, removed the pressure syringe, inserted and rotated the inner core needle.After about 3 ~ 5 minutes, pulled out the transfixion pin.These operation could ensure the needle not sticking together with the bone cement, and also could prevent the bone cement remaining in the transfixion pin because of premature pulling out.

Kept the patients remain in the prone position for 10 minutes or so.At the same time, observed the blood pressure, pulse and other vital signs without exception, turned over patients so that they were supine on a trolley and were transfered into the ward. Patients must continue to lie in bed for three days.Then they might get out of bed wearing abdominal belt. Routine antimicrobial drugs were used during surgery and 1 day after surgery ; generally 5 to 7 days later,the patients could discharge.

2.3 Follow-up method

Patients were taken the CT scan of vertebral compression fracture before operation to clear the posterior wall of vertebral body was integrity, and the filling condition of the bone cement in the vertebral body were observed again through CT scan of vertebral compression fracture after operation. At admission to hospital, preoperative, 3 days after operation, 1 month, 3 months, 6 months and 12 months after operation, taking the operative vertebral body as the center, the standand anteroposterior position and lateral poison thoracic or lumbar vertebrae X-ray were examined. Vertebral bodies height were measured using Vernier (central compression fracture, the central height was measured ; anterior border compression fracture, the anterior border height was measured,accurate to 0.1 mm).Then the loss rate of vetebral body height ,posterior salient angle, rectification rate of posterior salient angle ,VAS Score , antalgica usage score and locomotor activity score were observed at admission, preoperative, 3 days , 1 month , 3 months, 6 months and 12 months after operation.

2.3.1 Vertebral height measurement: The distance between the superior margin and the inferior margin in central part or leading edge of compressed vertebral body were measured.Then calculated the compressibility of vertebral height as follows: Using measurements from lateral X-rays, vertebral heights preoperative and postoperative could be found. Vertebral height lost = estimate of the original vertebral height - current height of the vertebral body, vertebral height loss rate (%) = loss of vertebral height / estimated original vertebral height x 100%.

2.3.2 Measurement methods of Kyphosis angle (Cobb angle): The vertical line of upper endplate on the upper vertebrae of the suffered and the vertical line of lower endplate on the lower vertebrae had a angle, that was the upper and lower endplate angle, reflecting the degree of the kyphosis severity. Calculating vertebral kyphosis correction rate in following way: In normal vertebral lateral X-ray, the upper endplate parallels to the lower.Vertebral kyphosis correction rate (%)=(preoperative vertebral kyphosis angle- postoperative vertebral kyphosis angle) / preoperative vertebral kyphosis angle.

2.3.3 VAS score: 0 point– turning round and coughing without pain; 1 point - quiet prostration without pain, coughing and turning round with pain ; 2 points - pain when coughing, deep breathing without pain; 3 points- lying without pain, coughing and deep breathing with pain; 4 points- quiet prostration with intermittent pain ; 5 points- quiet prostration with persistent pain; 6 points –quiet prostration with more pain; 7 points - severe pain, flip-flop and discomfort, being tired; 8 points – continuous, unbearable pain, sweating evidently all over the body; 9 points - severe unbearable pain accompanied by a sense of living death.

2.3.4 Analgesic usage score: 0 point: no usage of drugs; 1 point: use of non-steroidal anti-inflammatory drugs; 2 points: irregular use of narcotic analgesics; 3 points: regular usage of narcotic analgesics; 4 points: vein or muscle injections of narcotic analgesics.

2.3.5 Activity score: 1 point:acting without apparent difficulty; 2 points: difficulty walking and needing help; 3 points: only using a wheelchair or remain sitting; 4 points: being forced to lie in bed.

2.4 Statistical analysis

Numerical variables and ordinal variables were presented as mean ± standard deviation(SD).The vertabral height recovery rate and the Cobb angle correction rate were showed by percentage. Compared with the indicators at different time points by using SPSS11.0 for single-factor analysis of variance, A P value less than 0.05 was considered statistically significant.

3. Results

In this group of patients, the volume of bone cement injected in each vertebral was 3 ~ 6.5ml. When intraosseous vertebral venography were performed before the injection of bone cement, paravertebral vascular developed an image in 5 cases, then filled the gelatin sponge; peripheral cement leakage was found in 4 cases, intervertebral disc leakage was found in 2 cases and posterior margin leakage was seen in 2 cases (posterior longitudinal ligament is not exceeded), no clinical symptoms appeared. No nerve root or spinal cord injury,no pulmonary embolism or other complications were recorded. All patients had no further vertebral fractures. At admission,preoperative and postoperative X-ray films were shown in Figure 1-7. Figure 2 showed that bolster for self-replacement restored vertebral body height, corrected the kyphosis angle. Figure 5-7 showed that the PVP surgery could maintain and enhance the effect.The stata was showed in Table 1. Bolster for self-replacement combined with percutaneous vertebroplasty significantly improved VAS scores, analgesic use score and activity score, The results were shown in Table 2.

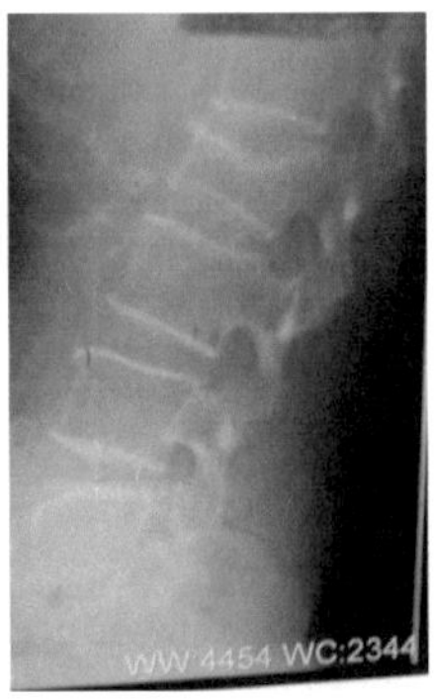

Fig. 1. Lateral X-ray at admission.

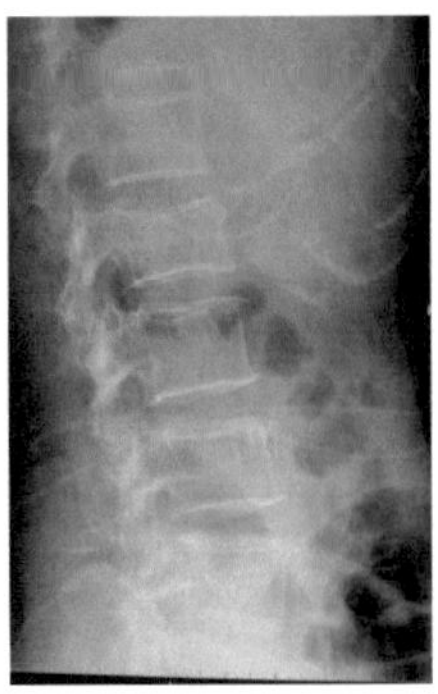

Fig. 2. Lateral X-ray before operation.

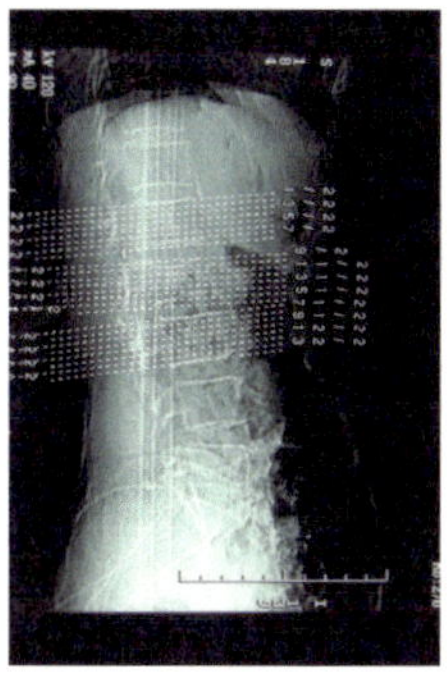

Fig. 3. Locating CT film before operation.

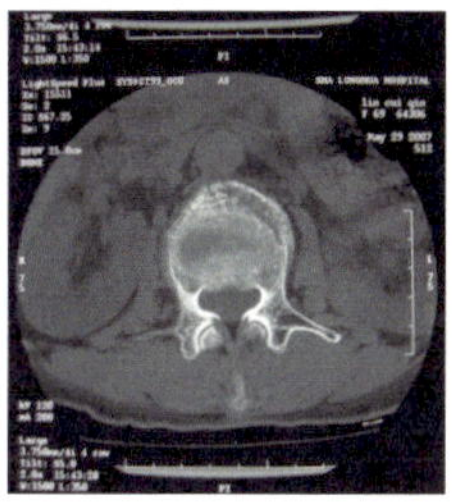

Fig. 4. CT plain scaning before operation.

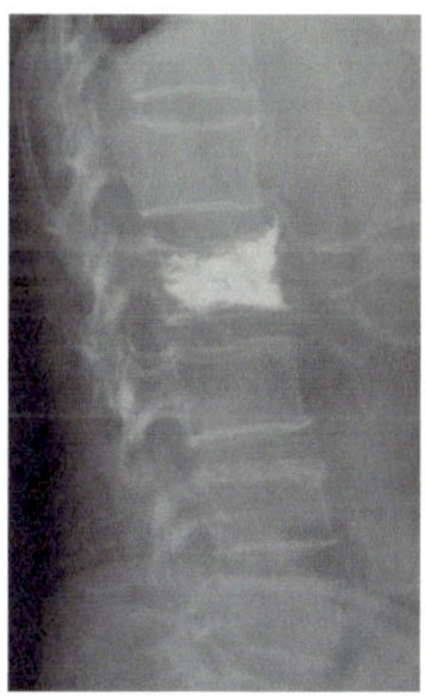

Fig. 5. Lateral X-ray after operation.

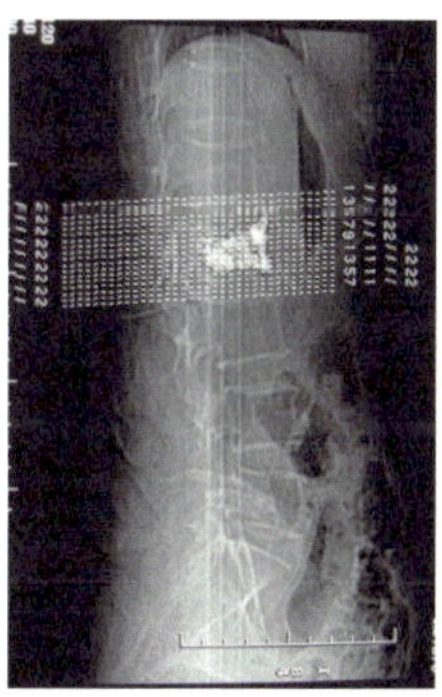

Fig. 6. Locating CT film after operation.

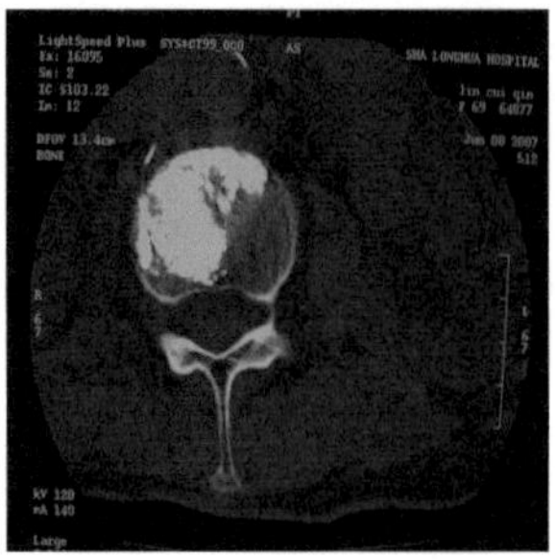

Fig. 7. CT plain scaning after operation.

Stage	Cases	Loss rate of vetebral body height	posterior salient angle	rectification rate of posterior salient angle
Admission	26	36.4 ±0.2	27.1 ±2.3	/
Pre-operating	26	8.4 ±0.2 #	11.2 ±2.2 #	58.7 ±1.5
3 days after operation	26	8.4 ±0.3 # *	9.9 ±1.9 # *	63.5 ±1.4*
1 month after operation	26	8.3 ±0.2 # *	9.8 ±1.8 # *	63.8 ±1.4*
3 months after operation	26	8.3 ±0.1 # *	9.9 ±2.2 # *	63.5 ±1.3*
6 months after operation	26	8.2 ±0.2 #*	9.7 ±2.2 #*	64.2 ±1.4*
1 year after operation	26	8.2 ±0.1 #*	9.7 ±2.3 #*	64.1 ±1.3*

Note:Comparing with admission, # P < 0.01; Different stages after operation comparing with each other and comparing with Pre-operating, *P > 0.05

Table 1. The results of loss rate of vetebral body height, posterior salient angle, rectification rate of posterior salient angle (x +s).

Stage	Cases	VAS Score	antalgica usage score	locomotor activity score
Admission	26	7.6± 0.02	1.4± 0.04	3.3± 0.02
Pre-operating	26	5.3± 0.02 △	1.3± 0.03 ▲	3.1± 0.01 ▲
3 days after operation	26	1.3± 0.01 △△	0.5± 0.04 △△	1.2± 0.03 △△
1 month after operation	26	0.3± 0.01 △△△★	0.1± 0.04 △△△★	1.1± 0.04 ★
3 months after operation	26	0.2± 0.01 △△△★	0.1± 0.03 △△△★	1.0± 0.02 ★
6 months after operation	26	0.1± 0.03 △△△★	0.1± 0.02 △△△★	1.0± 0.02 ★
1 year after operation	26	0.1± 0.02 △△△★	0.1± 0.01 △△△★	1.0± 0.03 ★

Note: VAS Score,comparing with admission, △P < 0.05. Antalgica usage score and locomotor activity score,Pre-operating comparing with admission, ▲ P > 0.05; 3 days after operation comparing with Pre-operating, △△P < 0.01. VAS Score and antalgica usage score, other stages after operation comparing witn 3 days after operation, △△△P < 0.01.locomotor activity score, other stages after operation comparing witn 3 days after operation, ★P > 0.05. 1 month after operation, 3 months after operation, 6 months after operation and 1 year after operation comparing with each other, P > 0.05.

Table 2. The results of VAS Score , antalgica usage score and locomotor activity score (x +s).

As could be seen from Table 1, in all cases after bolster for self-replacement, patients had a different degree of vertebral height restoration, and had significant differences compared with conditions at admission; vertebral height did not change significantly after PVP. Bolster for self-replacement was effective in restoring vertebral body height to compensate for the lack of PVP. Follow-up found no significant loss of vertebral height after surgery, indicating the effectiveness of PVP.

As could be seen from Table 2, although there were some recovery of vertebral height after bolster for self-replacement, that did not solve the problem of pain; After PVP, the patient's pain, activity had significantly improved, and these effects were stable in middle and long-term observation.

4. Discussion

4.1 Compressed vertebral body height restoration

Do not try to restore compression with PVP to normal vertebral body height [1]. The normal vertebral body height is the foundation of stable spine, when compression fractures occur, the trabeculars in the bone break, the breakage of cortical bone region occurs. When injecting bone cement during the plasty of the vertebral, it can have a good dispersion in the trabecular bone by applying appropriate pressure. But if we try to inject bone cement by larger pressure to restore vertebral height, the bone cement may have a leakage from the split to the vertebral surface, then flow into the peripheral of vertebral and canalis spinalis, causing neurological and vascular symptoms, fat embolism may also occur [2]. Xuyi[3] etc. considered that the injection volume of bone cement for thoracic and lumbar was 4 ~ 6ml,this dose had been able to achieve therapeutic purposes, the injection of large doses made it easy to cause vertebral body break and bone cement spillage, especially in elderly osteoporotic compression fractures.We should not be in the pursuit of simply increasing the amount of bone cement to improve the clinical effects of treatment. In addition,the compression level is more than 50% with instable fracture, PVP should be used with caution.

4.2 The choice of puncture site

As to unilateral or bilateral transpedicular percutaneous vertebroplasty, various reports are different. We believe that as long as the transfixion pin tip is just in the central of vertebral body in the anteroposterior and the anterior 1 / 3 in the lateral, most of the bone cement within vertebral fill well to the opposite side; what's more it is not that the more bone cement in vertebral body the better, so we have chosen unilateral transpedicular percutaneous vertebroplasty, it has obtained good clinical efficacy and also reduced the burden of patients.

4.3 Management of leakage of intravascular contrast agent showing

VCF, especially osteoporotic VCF, most blood sinus in the vertebral body communicates with the larger blood vessels outside the vertebral body.When PVP is carried out, bone cement may flow with blood flowing which leads to embolism in other parts. Thus, in contrast agent imaging, such as found in large vessels (diameter> 3mm) imaging, we should change the puncture site or choose contralateral puncture site, if this still cannot be avoided, it is best to abandon the surgery. If the contrast agent images in small vessels (diameter<3mm), fill the vertebral body with the gelatin sponge, pressing with a guide needle and then intraosseous vertebral venography should be performed again. If it is not obvious, we can continue to inject. For such patients, by increasing the viscosity of bone cement, inject bone cement of 0.5ml at first, wait for 2-3minutes and then adopt the slow injection method, which allows the formation of lumps of bone cement to block transport vessels, to avoid the infiltration of blood vessels and embolism that may be caused further.

4.4 Control of bone cement viscosity

The bone cement viscosity can be controlled by adjusting the ratio of powder and liquid during the surgery. For serious osteoporosis, the magnitude of the contrast agent widely distributed in the vertebral body, or vascular imaging, the bone cement viscosity should be increased; on the contrary,the bone cement viscosity should be reduced to enable better diffusion in the vertebral body.

4.5 Notice

Because there is still 0.5ml bone cement in the transfixion needle tubing, when we insert inner core needle at the end ,the bone cement will get into the vertebral body too.So when the bone cement get close to the hinder margin of vertebral body(<1 mm)in the surgery, inserting must be stopped to prevent the leakage of bone cement.

In recent years, surgical techniques tend to be minimally invasive, that's to say, minimize iatrogenic trauma to a minimum in order to obtain the desired effect[4]. PVP has the advantages such as less trauma, shorter operative time, obvious analgetic effect, rapid postoperative recovery and so on, especially for elderly osteoporotic patients,it has less systemic interference and higher security, patients can have ambulation as early as possible to avoid leading to complications because of prolonged bed rest, therefore, it has broad application prospects. But its long-term clinical efficacy remains to be observed.

Moreover, PMMA which is the earliest and most widespread used in clinic has the disadvantages such as heart and pulmonary toxicity, heat production, leakage and so on.Some researchers have tried to use biodegradable Calcium acid phosphate bone cement(CPC) and calcium phosphate bone cement/bone morphogenetic protein (CPC/BMP)with bone conduction and tissue compatibility to replace PMMA. However, animal experiments have found that [5],CPC and CPC / BMP can't restore the strength and stiffness of the vertebral body well in the near future , it is not conducive to osteoporotic vertebral compression fracture healing, therefore it can not completely replace PMMA. So PMMA is the mainly filler in application now[6]. It is believed that with the development of science and technology, especially the development of biological materials science, safer and more rational fillings are bound to come out in the future[7].

5. Comparative study between vertebroplasty using bolster technique and balloon kyphoplasty

Simple PVP treatment can not recover the losed height of the vertebral, balloon kyphoplasty (PKP) are developing at recent years. Part 1 to part 4 indicated that bolster for self-replacement combined with PVP had good clinical effect in treatment of vertebral compression fractures.In order to compare the curative effects between bolster for self-replacement combined with PVP and PKP,this study was underwent.

6. Materials and methods

6.1 Bolster for self-replacement combined with PVP

The clinical materials and therapeutic methods were uniformity with Part 1 to part 4.

6.2 PKP

Clinical materials

There were 18 men and 67 women in the 85 cases of VCF studied. Ages ranged from 47 to 94 years, with a mean of 75.03±9.77years. All cases had no neurological symptoms or signs of root damage. Pre-operative CR and CT scans of vertebra showed a complete posterior vertebral body.

Therapeutic methods

The operation was carried out under the surveillance of the C-arm, Thoracic and lumbar punctures were achieved through the lateral neck of vertebral. An anteroposterior fluoroscopy C-arm tube was used to adjust the angle, so that both lateral neck of vertebrals showed clearly, two Kirschner wires crossed and were fixed on the skin surface, the surface projection of lateral vertebral neck coincided with the intersection of the two Kirschner wires.The puncture point lay slightly outside and above,1 ~ 1.5cm from the coincidence point. After local anesthesia, the transfixion pin and body sagittal appeared 15 ° ~ 30 ° angle,after the transfixion pin got into the lateral vertebral neck, then pushed the transfixion pin 1 ~ 2cm. Checking under lateral fluoroscopy to confirm correct transfixion point,Penetrated with slow rotation, so that the transfixion pin tip was in the central of vertebral body in the anteroposterior and the anterior 1 / 3 in the lateral;After reaming with hollow drill, gelatin sponge were filled, then balloon dilatation catheter was inserted slowly to anteroposterior and the anterior 1 / 3 of the vertebtal body,pressurizing gradually. Vertebral bodies height recovered under the surveillance of the C-arm,balloon dilatation catheter exited.Then injected 4~6 mL cement into the vertebral body under fluoroscopy.When bone cement was near the posterior margin of the vertebral body,stopped pushing.

After injection, removed the pressure syringe, inserted and rotated the inner core needle.After about 3 ~ 5 minutes, pulled out the transfixion pin.These operation could ensure the needle not sticking together with the bone cement, and also could prevent the bone cement remaining in the transfixion pin because of premature pulling out.

6.3 Observed indexes

VAS Score,antalgica usage score, Oswestry disability index of functional, Cobb angle were observed pre-operation and 3 months after operation.Cement leakages were observed in the operation.

6.4 Statistical analysis

Numerical variables and ordinal variables were presented as mean ± standard deviation(SD).The cement percolation rate were showed by percentage. Compared with the indicators by using SPSS18.0 for single-factor analysis of variance, A P value less than 0.05 was considered statistically significant.

7. Results

The statistical analysis were not statistically significant in the curative effects between bolster for self-replacement combined with PVP and PKP, the stata was showed in Table 3. The cement percolation rate of PKP was lower than that of bolster for self-replacement combined with PVP, the stata was showed in Table 4. Preoperative and postoperative X-ray films of PKP were shown in Figure 8-9.

Methods	Cases	VAS Score		antalgica usage score		Oswestry disability index		Cobb's angle	
		pre	post	pre	post	pre	post	pre	post
PVP	26	5.30± 0.02	0.2± 0.01*	1.30± 0.03	0.10± 0.03*	42.15± 0.89	8.96± 1.38*	11.20± 2.20	9.9 0± 2.10**
PKP	85	6.77± 1.27##	0.19± 0.98*#	1.73± 0.45##	0.15± 0.048*#	41.88± 1.24#	9.08± 1.16*#	21.14± 1.49###	9.76± 1.48*#

Note:Comparing with pre-operation, * P < 0.01, ** P >0.05; Comparing with PVP using bolster, # P >0.05, ## P<0.05, ### P<0.0.1

Table 3. The curative effects between PVP using bolster and PKP (x +s).

Methods	Cases	Percolation cases	percolation rate (%)	Cobb's angle before operation	Cement quantity (ml)
PVP	26	13	50.0	11.15±2.51	4.52±0.75
PKP	85	11	12.9###	21.15±1.49###	4.43±1.11#

Note: Comparing with PVP using bolster, ### P<0.0.1, # P >0.05.

Table 4. The cement percolation rate between PVP using bolster bolster and PKP.

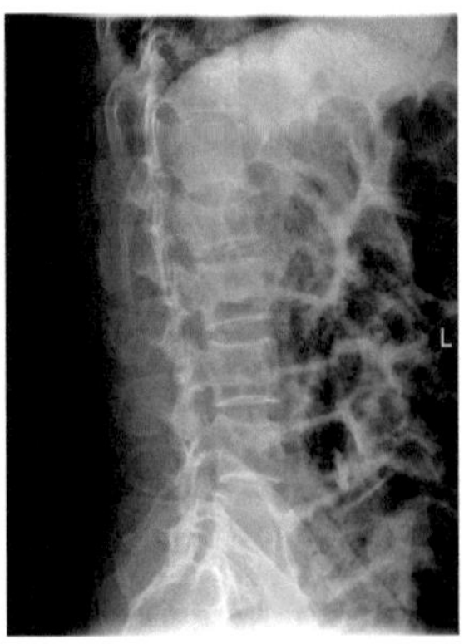

Fig. 8. Lateral X-ray before PKP.

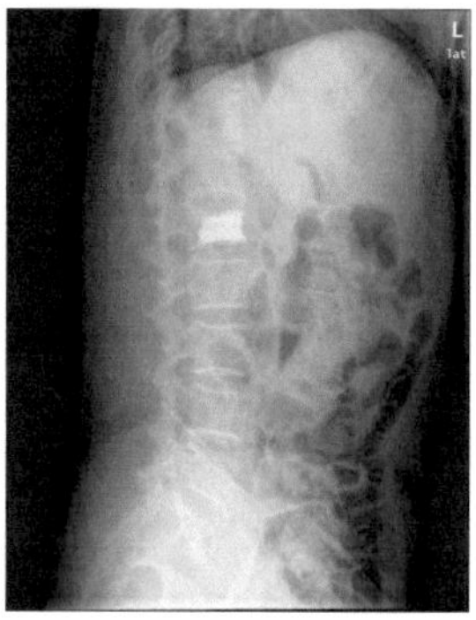

Fig. 9. Lateral X-ray afterr PKP.

8. Discussion

8.1 The role of bolster for self-replacement

As simple PVP treatment can not recover the losed height and has leakage or other shortcomings, balloon kyphoplasty (percutaneous kyphoplasty,PKP) has appeared in recent years. Although PKP can increase vertebral body height, and also reduce the leakage of bone cement into the vessel,therefore avoiding the formation of thrombosis[8], it has some disadvantages. For example, it cannot control the direction of expansion and the compliance of the balloons in the vertebral body are not good enough , there is a 20% balloon rupture rate in the expansion process, it can only used for fresh fractures[9], while the price is relatively more expensive and many patients cannot afford. No balloon rupture appeared in our study,it maybe because of that the sample size is not large.

While PKP is more relatively difficult than PVP in the operation, so PKP is subject to certain restrictions in the application. Therefore, PVP is still the most common method for VCF treatment. The restorations of thoracic and lumbar height mainly rely on the reposition of body position. The device resetting plays a role on the basis of reposition of body position and the main role is to maintain reduction [10]. So before the operation we can restore the vertebral height gradually by traditional measures such as lying on the back on hard wood bed with a bostler under the back and "five-point support method" which exercises lumbar-back muscular function (typically the recovery happens in 3 to 5 days , without the formation of trabecular malunion), then take the PVP treatment to compensate for the weakness in restoring vertebral height.

In addition, we used the method reported by some literatures [11] that bone cement should be placed at -4 °C refrigerator for 5 ~ 10minutes before operation to extend the operating time, thereby reducing the incidence of complications and obtained good efficacy.In spite of with 50% cement percolation rate,no clinical symptoms were observed.

8.2 The curative effects between PVP using bolster and PKP

Simple PVP treatment can not recover the losed height of the vertebral body[12]. Bolster for self-replacement can recover the losed height of the vertebral body before PVP. So PVP using bolster has the same effects comparing with PKP on reducing VAS Score,antalgica usage score, Oswestry disability index of functional, Cobb's angle[13].Because we found that the effects of PVP using bolster have been stable from 3 months after operation,so we only compare the indexes before operation and 3 months after operation between PVP using bolster and PKP.

Because PVP using bolster has 50% cement percolation rate and balloon kyphoplasty has lower percolation rate(12.9%), broken instable VCF should be treated by balloon kyphoplasty first.

9. References

[1] Tan ZJ, Xu JZ, Zhou Q. Experience and key point in vertebroplasty. J Trauma Surg, 2005,7:347-348.

[2] Koessler MJ, Ebli N, Pitto RP. Fat and bone marrow embolism during percutaneous vertebroplasty. Anesth Analg, 2003,97:293.

[3] Xu Y, Liu YJ, Dong Y. Classification, prevention and treatment of bone cement leakage following percutaneous ventebraplasty. J Fourth Mil Med Univ, 2006, 27: 155-157.

[4] Wu Zhenping, Cheng Shaodan, Yang Hao, et al. Clinical research progress in interventional therapy of femoral head necrosis. J Tradi Chin Orthop and Trauma, 2003,15:630-631.

[5] Li D, Yin YS, Liu W, et al. Experimental study on the different injectable material in vertebroplaety. Chin Remedies & Clinics,2005,6(3):175-178.

[6] Cheng Shao-dan, Mo Wen, Hu Zhi-jun, et al. Bone cement infusion and complications during percutaneous vertebroplasty. Journal of Clinical Rehabilitative Tissue Engineering Research.2009,13(8):1593-1596

[7] Mo Wen, Cheng Shaodan, Hu Zhijun, et al. The research on bolster for self-replacement combined with percutaneous vertebroplasty in treatment of vertebral compression fractures. Chinese Journal of Osteoporosis,2008,14(12):903-907

[8] Coumans JV, Reinhardt MK, Lieberman IH. Kyphoplasty for vertebral compression fractures: 1 year clinical outcomes from aprospective study. J Neurosurg, 2003,99(1S):44-50.

[9] Lieberman IH, Dudeney S, Reinhardt MK, et al. Initial outcome and efficacy of kyphoplasty in the treatment of painful osteoporotic vertebral compression fracture. Spine,2001,26:1631-1638.

[10] Ma Yz, Zhen ZG. Clinical Internal Fixation of Bone. Anhui Science and technology publishing house,1999:348-349.

[11] Cheng Shaodan, Mo Wen, Shi Qi, et al. Research progress in percutaneous vertebroplasty curing vertebral fracture. Chinese Journal of Osteoporosis, 2007, 13(12):879-883.

[12] Marek Szpalski, Robert Gunzburg. Vertebral Osteoporotic Compression Fracture. Lippincott Williams & Wikins, U.S.A, 2003.

[13] Yu Zhixing, Mo Wen, Ma Junming, et al. A retrospective analysis about 111 cases of PVP/PKP in the treatment of thoracolumbar osteoporotic fractures. Chinese Journal of Osteoporosis, 2011,17(9):26-31.

Part 2

Minimally Invasive Spinal Surgery

5

Minimally Invasive Extreme Lateral Trans-Psoas Approach to the Lumbar Spine: Applications and Techniques

Brian Hood and Steven Vanni
University of Miami, Miller School of Medicine, Jackson Memorial Hospital, Miami, FL
USA

1. Introduction

The biomechanical advantages to a load sharing anterior lumbar construct have not been debated. The development of a technique to place such a construct has gone through an evolution through PLIF, to open ALIF, to endoscopic ALIF. Recently the technique of a direct lateral mini-open approach has been popularized through the development of better retraction, improved visibility, and superior results. In the following chapter, we describe the technique, the indications, and the potentials for complications that surgeons need to comprehend before employing this powerful tool.

2. History

Historically, spine surgery was performed through a posterior approach as it was the most direct pathway to the bony structures. Anterior approaches to the spine were initially developed in response tuberculosis. An anterior approach to the treatment of spondylolisthesis was first reported by Burns in 1933[1]. Since its first description, anterior lumbar interbody surgery has been used for the treatment of spinal deformity, spinal instability, tumors, infection and chronic low back pain including "failed back syndrome"[2-4] In 1953 Cloward[5] described performing an interbody fusion from a posterior approach which allowed a complete decompression of the neural elements as we as performing a 360 degree fusion without violating the abdominal viscera and retroperitoneal structures.

In the 1970's , despite satisfactory results from multiple authors, the anterior approach was condemned for causing undue surgical trauma to the patient with a considerable complication rate as well as postoperative morbidity[6].

The laproscopic ALIF was developed as a minimally invasive alternative to the traditional ALIF and mini-open ALIF and has been reported to be a safe surgical procedure[7]. Laparoscopic procedures still share some complications of open surgery such as great vessel injury, retrograde ejaculation, and arterial thromboembolism [8-10]. In addition to the morbidity of open anterior surgery, laparoscopy introduces its own set of challenges such as bowel injury during the percutaneous approach, CO2 insufflation leading to low cardiac output [11]. In addition, depth perception is compromised with two dimensional imaging and most neurosurgeons are unfamiliar with the use of laparoscopic instruments. Regardless of mini-open or laparoscopic, access to the anterior lumbar spine is still dependent on a competent general or vascular surgeon. Biomechanical insufficiency of the ventral lumbar spine is still a common clinical problem for spine surgeons and the ability to access and intervene is an important tool in ones surgical armamentarium.

In searching for ways to improve patient care and reduce operative morbidity there have been many significant improvements in instrumentation and technique. Minimally invasive techniques have evolved over the ensuing decade and now encompass all aspects of lumbar spine surgery. The advantages of minimal access surgery include minimal tissue disruption leading to a decrease in postoperative pain and more rapid post operative mobilization. In addition, decreased disruption of the paraspinal muscles and ligaments allows for proper maintenance of spinal biomechanics. Advances in retractors and instrumentation allow direct access to the site of pathology decreasing the size of exposure for many procedures.

The anterolateral approach first reported for the treatment of Potts disease was adapted to the treatment of throacolumbar fractures by McAfee[12]. Mayer reported a minimally invasive retroperitoneal microscopic approach for access to L2-L5 in patients having undergone previous posterior procedures[13]. McAffe later reported an endoscopic procedure that involved balloon dissection of the retrotransversalis fascia and allowed placement of an interbody device [14].

The application of tubular retractors to lumbar surgery contributed significantly to the advancement of minimally invasive spinal surgery. In 1998, the METRx-MD (Medtronic Sofamor Danek, Memphis, TN) was introduced allowing the use of the intraoperative microscope in addition to the edoscope. The fixed tube was modified to a split blade design that could accommodate a microscope, or by the use of fiberoptic light, loupe magnification.

Bergey reported an endoscopic transpsoas approach for the treatment of degenerative scoliosis [15]. Pimenta described a minimally invasive transpsoas retroperitoneal approach using tubular retractors, and in doing so allowed spine surgeons to have access to the power of an anterior approach through a minimally invasive route that didn't require an access surgeon [16].

The XLIF approach to the anterior spinal column has some distinct advantages over traditional anterior and posterior approaches.

- A true minimally invasive approach involving minimal disruption of tissues resulting in less blood loss, decreased postoperative pain, and a shorter recovery time.
- Surgical exposure is adequate, safe and reproducible.
- Avoids disruption, destruction, and denervation of posterior musculature.
- Preserves the posterior ligamentous complex (PLC) allowing preserved anatomical load sharing, motion coupling, stability, and facilitates alignment and decompression via ligamentotaxis.
- Avoids iatrogenic instability via resection of the posterior bony elements.
- Decreased risk of vascular injury.
- Surgical access to the disc space allows for a thorough disc removal and endplate preparation.
- Maximized access to the ring apophysis supporting axial and coronal deformity correction and facilitation of alignment.

2.1 Biomechanics, indications and contraindications

Biomechanically, the lateral interbody fusion is a minimally invasive, muscle and ligament sparing procedure that allows preservation of the spine's inherent biomechanical stabilizers. Anterior column fusions provide a superior biomechanical environment for fusion. White and Panjabi evaluated the spinal ligamentous tensile strength and found the ALL to be the strongest ligament in the spine[17]. The biomechanics of a construct not only reflect the construct itself, but the approach to implant the construct. The traditional ALIF resects the ALL, and the PLIF and TLIF resect a varying degree of the posterior elements. The size or "footprint" of the interbody implant as well as its position within the interspace also influences the biomechanics of the construct. The large lateral interbody spans the ring apophysis and provides maximum vertebral support.

The surgical indications for the extreme lateral interbody fusion is essentially any thoracolumbar case above L5-S1 requrinig access to the disc space and/or vertebral bodies. We will focus more on individual pathologies throughout the chapter, but as an overview:

- Degenerative disc disease (DDD) with instability.
  - The benefits of using an extreme lateral interbody fusion for DDD include stabilization of the affected level with restoration of the disc space height. In doing so, an indirect decompression of the neural foramina is seen as restoring the disc height leads to significantly increased foraminal volume.
- Recurrent disc herniation.
  - Using a lateral access corriodor allows the surgeon to avoid scar tissue, adequately decompress the neural elements, and perform a fusion all through a minimal access corridor.
- Degenerative spondylolisthesis.
  - Because the anterior and posterior longitudinal ligament remain intact, listhesis can be relieved through ligamentotaxis. In addition, because of the exposure obtained through a lateral portal, a much larger interbody graft can b e placed thatn those used with standard posterior lumbar interbody (PLIF) or transforaminal lumbar interbody fusion (TLIF).
- Degenerative scoliosis.
  - Extreme lateral trans-psoas approach is able to provide the benefits of both the ALIF and PLIF/TLIF techniques and minimize the negative aspects.
- Pseudoarthrosis
  - The lateral access corridor minimizes dissection through previous scar tissue and allows the placement of a large interbody graft under compression allowing for improved stability after a failed posterior fusion.
- Discitis, Osteomyelitis.
  - The exposure provide allows for a thorough discectomy and cleaning of the endplates.
- Total disc replacement (TDR)revision
  - Lateral access allows a large TDR implant to be removed without compromising the neural elements or having to reexplore the anterior exposure at levels above L5-S1.
- Post laminectomy instability, deformity

    - Iatrogenic deformity created by multilevel laminectomies is an ideal situation for lateral access for correction of the deformity through restoration of anterior height, providing a stable fusion, as well as avoiding complications of revision surgery.
- Junctional disease
    - We frequently employ the Lateral route for patients who have failed either above or below previous constructs.

Several limitations merit discussion prior to considering a lateral approach to pathology.

- Anomalous vascular anatomy interfering with the lateral approach.
    - When dealing with idiopathic scoliosis with severe rotational deformities, the coronal and saggital rotations may lead to vascular structures impeding lateral access. Careful scrutiny of preoperative MRI is imperative to preventing complications.
- Bilateral retroperitoneal scarring.
    - A history of nephrectomy or other retroperitoneal surgery precludes safe access on the side of previous pathology. A history of anterior lumbar interbody fusion (ALIF) or previous lateral approach are not absolute contraindications to lateral access.
- Degenerative spondylolistheis of grade III or greater.
    - In high grade spondylolisthesis t he exiting nerve root is located in a more anterior position. In addition, it is difficult to find the anatomical center to place the interbody graft.
- Cannot access L5-S1
    - Some surgeons will resect a portion of the iliac crest, in general though, the L5-S1 level is best addressed with a PLIF/TLIF.
- Renal cysts, or the presence of a horseshoe kidney may preclude lateral access.

2.2 Anatomy

The retroperitoneal space is the area of the posterior abdominal wall located between the posterior parietal peritoneum and the posterior part of the transversalis fascia (Figure 1). The adrenal glands, kidneys and ureters are located in the retroperitoneal space as well as lumbar plexus, the aorta, and the inferior vena cava and their tributaries.

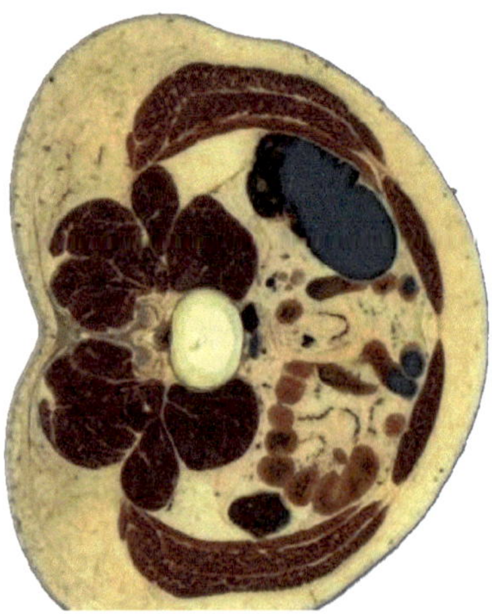

Fig. 1. Axial illustration of patient oriented for retroperitoneal transpsoas access to the lumbar spine.

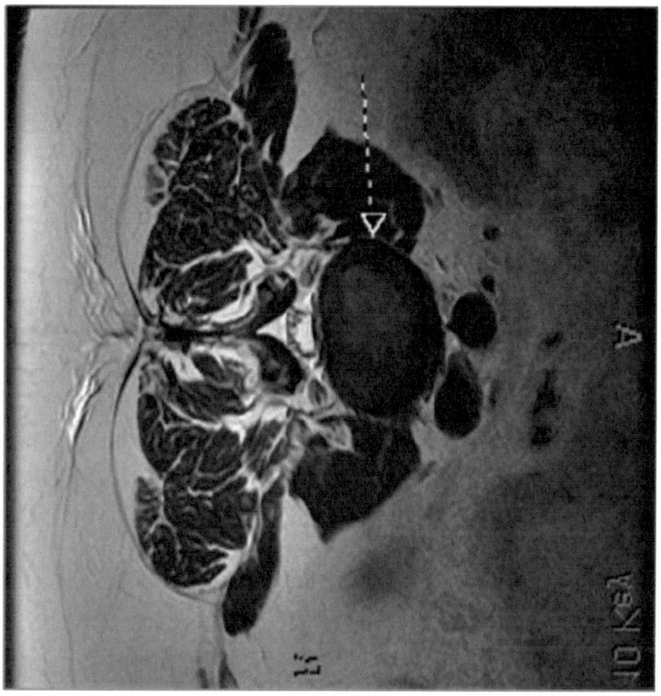

Fig. 2. MRI oriented in anatomical position for retroperitoneal transpsoas access to the lumbar spine.

The anterior and lateral abdominal muscles include the obliques (external and internal), the transverses abdominis, and rectus abdominus. After dissection through the skin and subcutaneous tissue, the first muscular layer, and most superficial is the external oblique. After passing through the external oblique, the next muscle encountered is the internal oblique. The only two structures passing through the internal and external oblique muscles are the iliohypogastric and illioinguinal branches of L1, both are purely sensory brances. Immediately under the internal oblique is the transversalis muscle. The final muscle transvered during the approach is the psoas major. The muscle originates from tendinous arches between vertebra diminishing in size as it traverses the pelvic brim, and fuctions as a hip flexor, abductor and lateral rotator. The lumbar plexus lies within the substance of the psoas major (Figure 2 with arrow passing through the psoas major). The genitofemoral nerve can be visualized on the anterior surface of the muscle.

Four paired lumbar arteries emerge from the posterior aspect of the aorta (Figure 3). The venous supply runs with the arteries draining into the vena cava. The bifurcation the aorta and vena cava into the common iliac vessels generally occurs around the L4-5 disc space. Targeting the center of the disc space generally avoids contact with the anteriorly placed vasculature. The location of blood vessels is shown below (Figures 4-7).

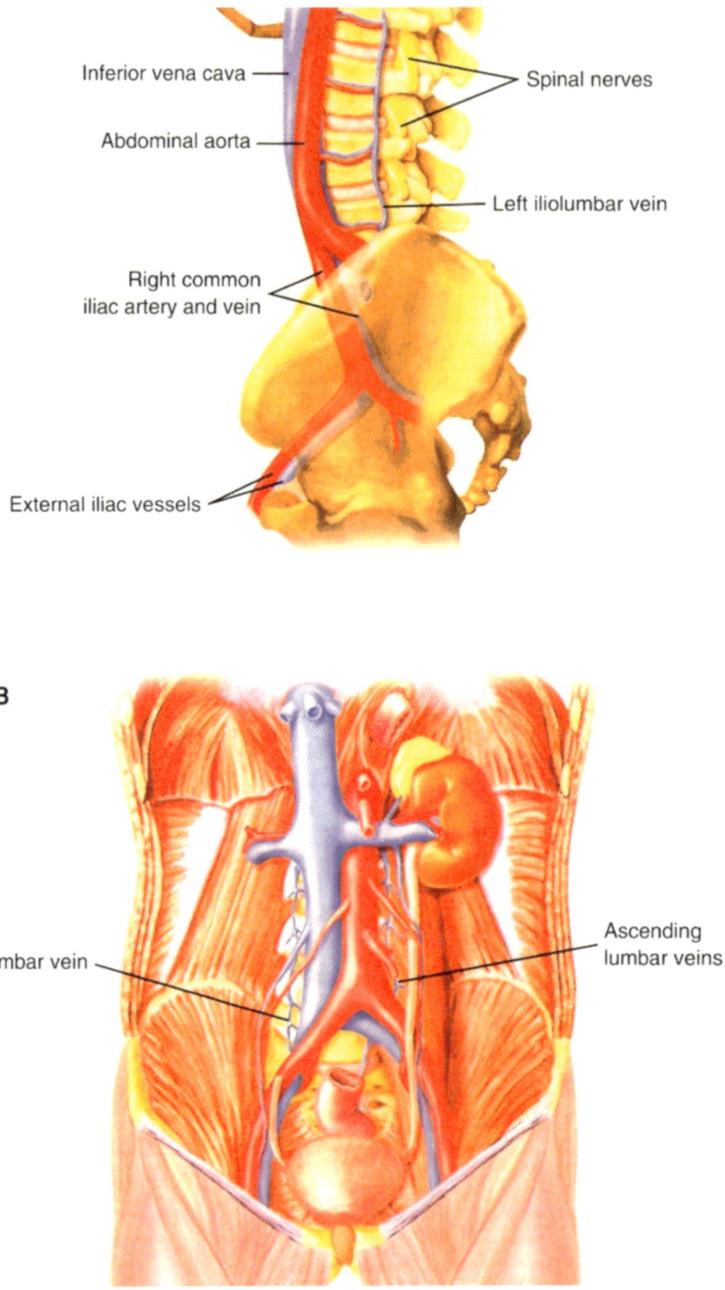

Fig. 3. The major lumbar vasculature.

L1-2 BLOOD VESSEL LOCATIONS

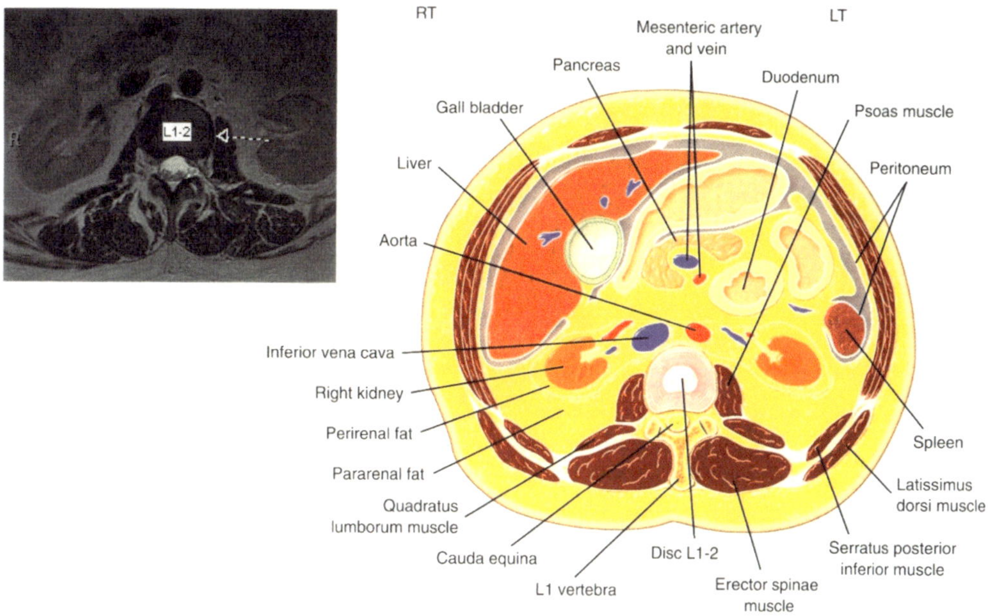

Fig. 4. L1-2 Blood vessel locations.

L2-3 BLOOD VESSEL LOCATIONS

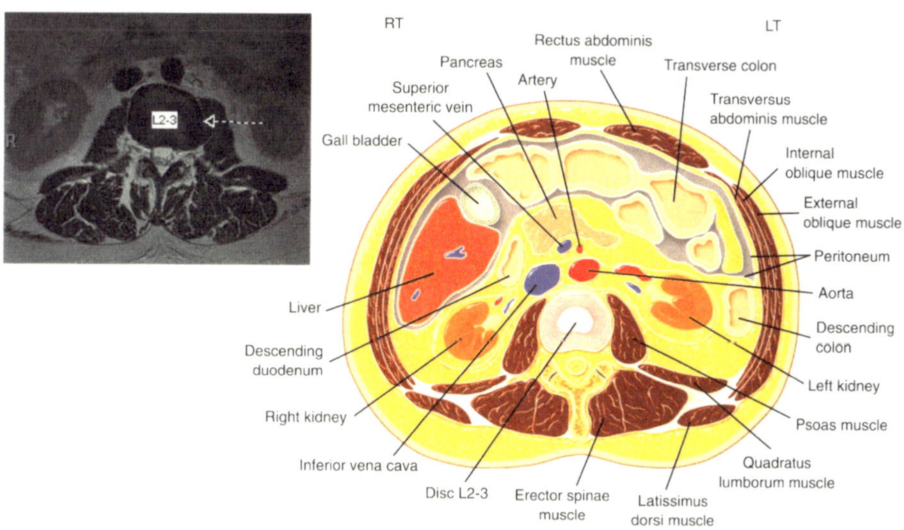

Fig. 5. L2-3 Blood vessel locations.

L3-4 BLOOD VESSEL LOCATIONS

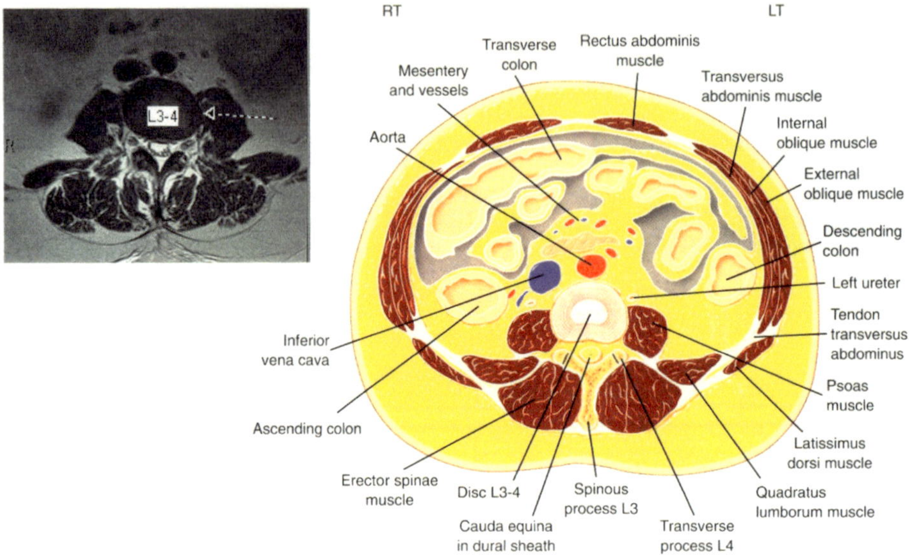

Fig. 6. L3-4 Blood vessel locations.

L4-5 BLOOD VESSEL LOCATIONS

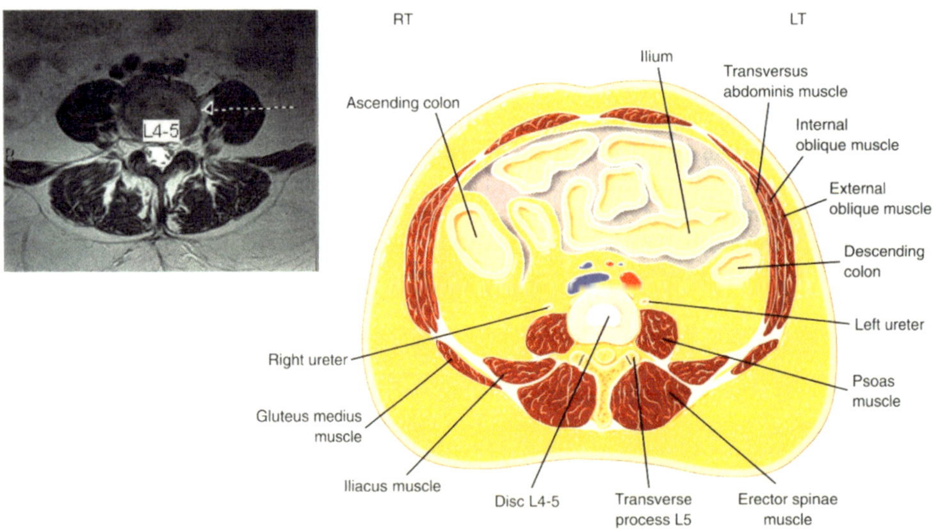

Fig. 7. L4-5 Blood vessel locations.

The Lumbar Plexus

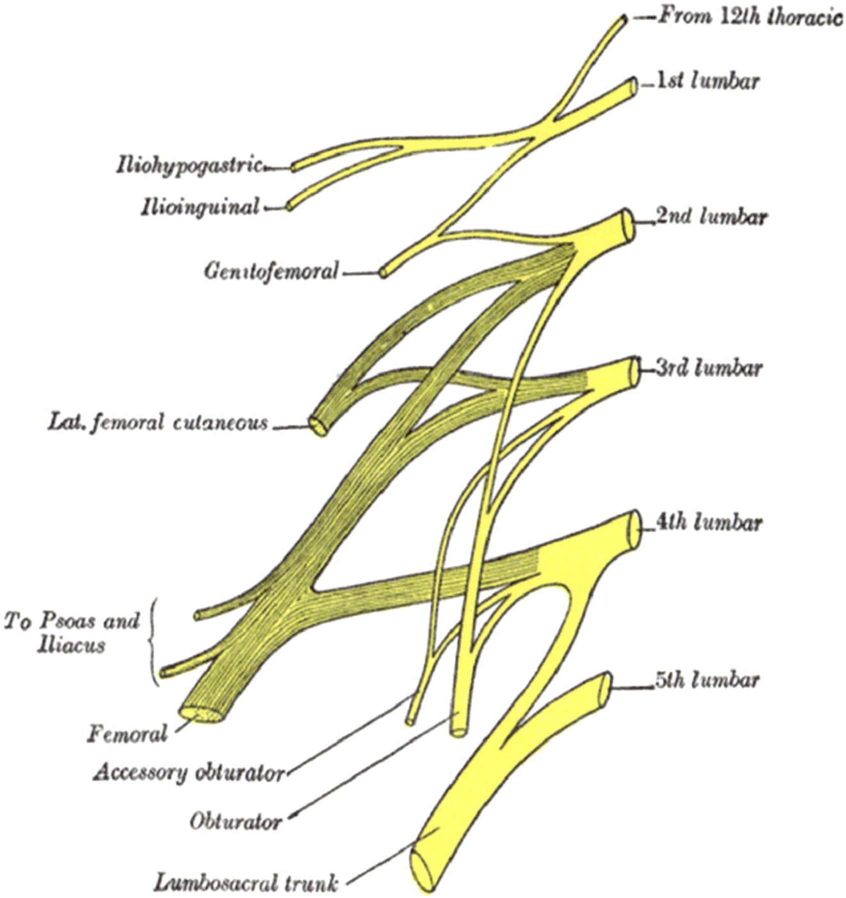

Fig. 8. The lumbar plexus.

The lumbar plexus is formed by the ventral rami of the first three lumbar roots and part of the foruth root and is generally located in the posterior substance of the psoas muscle (Figure 8). L1 gives off the iliohypogastric and ilioinguinal nerves which travel superficially through the retroperitoneal space and then pass to run between the internal and external obliques and supply sensation to the groin. L1 and L2 both contribute to the genitofemoral nerve which lies on the anterior fascia of the psoas muscle and provides sensation to the genital and femoral regions. L2 and L3 give rise to the lateral cutaneous nerve of the thigh wich innervates the anterolateral and lateral surfaces of the thigh. The large femoral nerve receives contributions from L2, L3 and L4 lies within the psoas muscle and innervates the quadriceps muscles. The obturator nerve innervates the adductor muscles of the thigh and provides cutaneous sensation to the inner thigh and receives contributions from L2, L3, L4 and exits at the medial border of the psoas and crosses the sacral ala.

In an anatomic survey, Benglis et al sought to delineate the location of the lumbar contributions to the lumbosacral plexus in relation to the respective disc spaces relevant to the transpsoas approach as seen via fluoroscopic imaging (L1-5)(Figures 9-11). The findings of their study suggested that the lumbosacral plexus migrates from a dorsal to ventral location from the L1 through the L5 disc spaces. Therefore, when targeting the center of the disc space for an extreme lateral procedure, the neural structures are at greatest risk of injury at the L4/5 level with a posteriorly positioned dilator or retractor. They also concluded that the risks of injuring inherent motor nerve branches directed to the posas muscle still exists even with neuromonitoring as well as injury to the genitofemoral nerve which pierces the psoas muscle and travels caudally on its ventral surface (at L1-2) supplying sensory innervations to the femoral triangle and creamasteric muscles in males).

Moro et al studied the configuration of the lumbar plexus in regard to the safety of the endoscopic transpsoas approach. After identifying the anterior and posterior borders of the vertebral body, they divided them into zones with zone 1 located anteriorly and zone IV located adjacent to the posterior margin of the vertebral body. They found that the most anterior position of the nerve was zone III and this was found at L4/5, and concluded that the safety zone should be L4/5 and above.

To prevent lumbosacral plexus injury a thorough understanding of the neural anatomy at various disc levels is essential. In addition, intraoperative monitorin is used. This includes free-run EMG and dynamic triggered EMP. This provides real time nerve proximity measurements that are critical to avoiding nerve injury during the transpsoas approach.

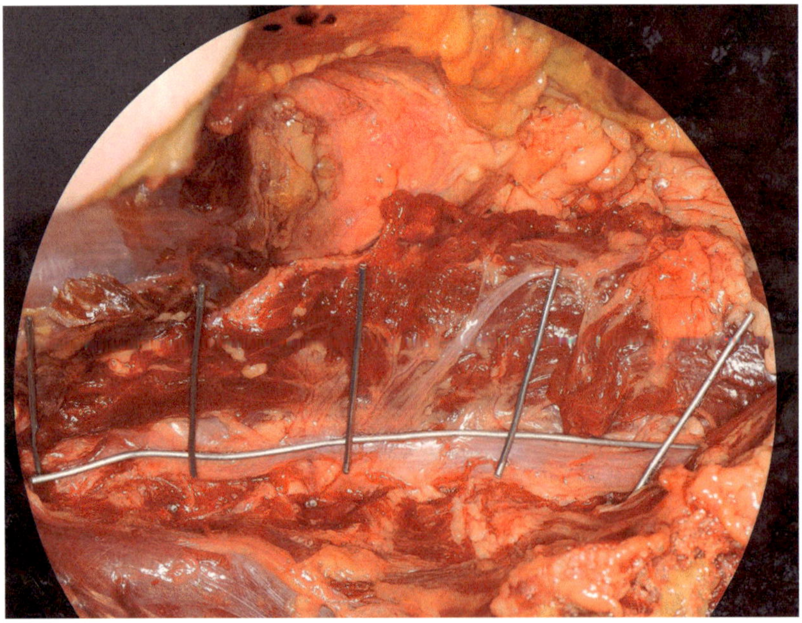

Fig. 9. Anatomical dissection with radiolucent markers placed on femoral nerve and over disc spaces.

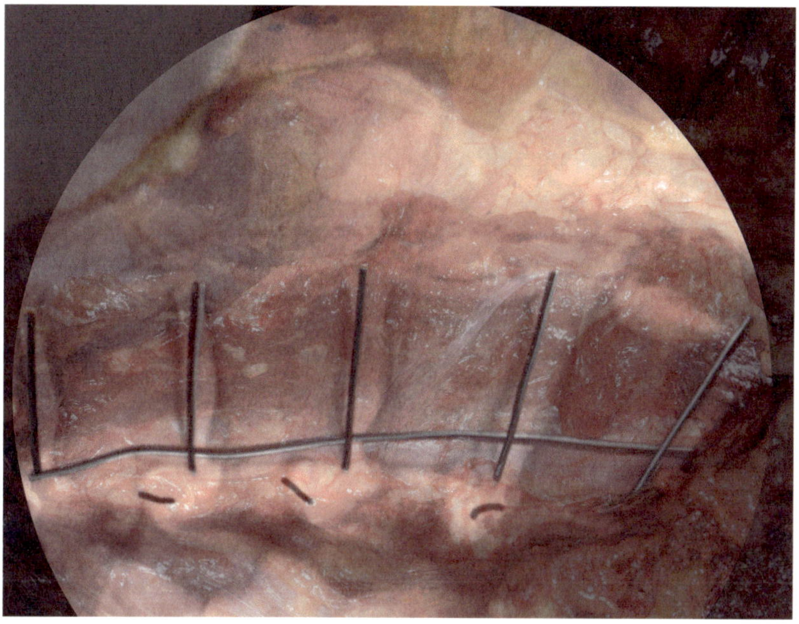

Fig. 10. Anatomical dissection with musculature removed with radiolucent markers over femoral nerve and disc spaces.

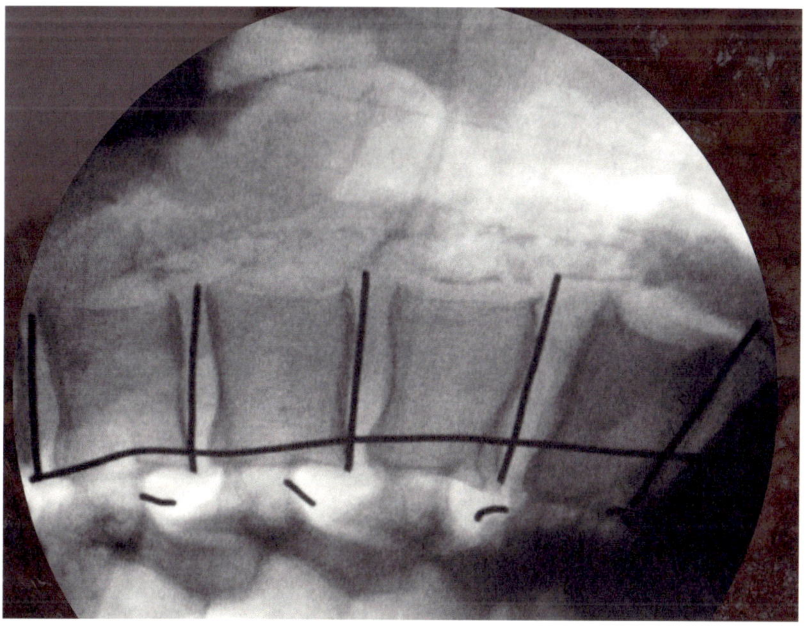

Fig. 11. Radiograph of anatomical dissection with radiolucent markers over the femoral nerve, the disc spaces, and in the respective foramen.

2.3 Summary

- The lumbar plexus was found within the psoas muscle lying predominately in a cleft at the junction of the transverse process and the vertebral body.
- There was a dorsal to ventral migration of the plexus in the lateral fluoroscopic view from L1 to L5.
- The plexus below L5 continued as the femoral nerve.
- The dilators and retractor should pass through the anterior portion of the psoas muscle and lie on the middle to anterior portion of the disc space.
- This is most relevant to the lateral approach at L4/5 (Figure 12).
- The use of free run EMG and discreet dynamic triggered EMG is essential, but its use can still result in nerve injury from compression via the retractor.
- The risk of sensory nerve injury is still present during this approach.

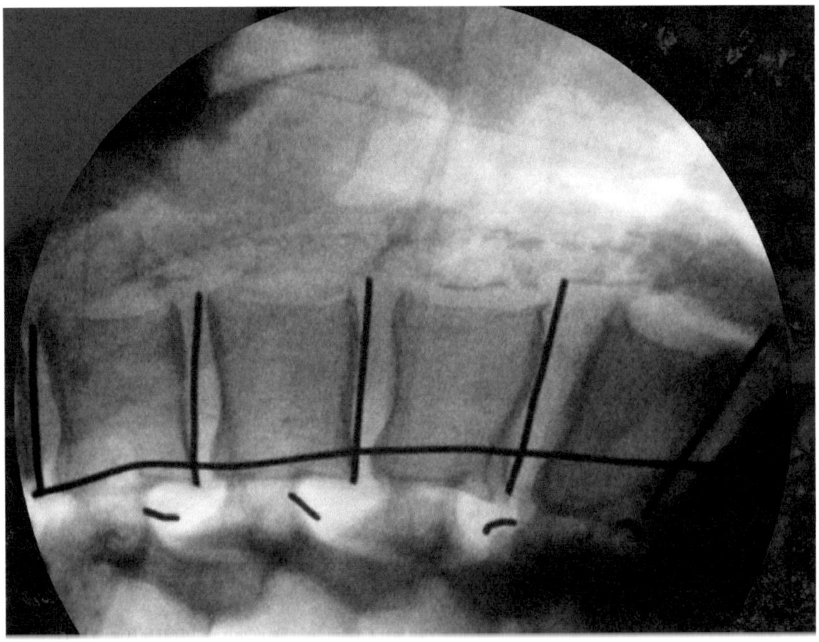

Fig. 12. Illustration of the risk of femoral nerve injury when attempting an L4-5 or L5-S1 lateral interbody fusion.

2.4 The approach

Performing a successful transpsoas procedure starts with the patient positioning and ensuring that adequate radiological visualization is possible. The operative table must be converted to the "reverse" orientation by replacing the head piece from the end above the base to the opposite side (Figure 13).

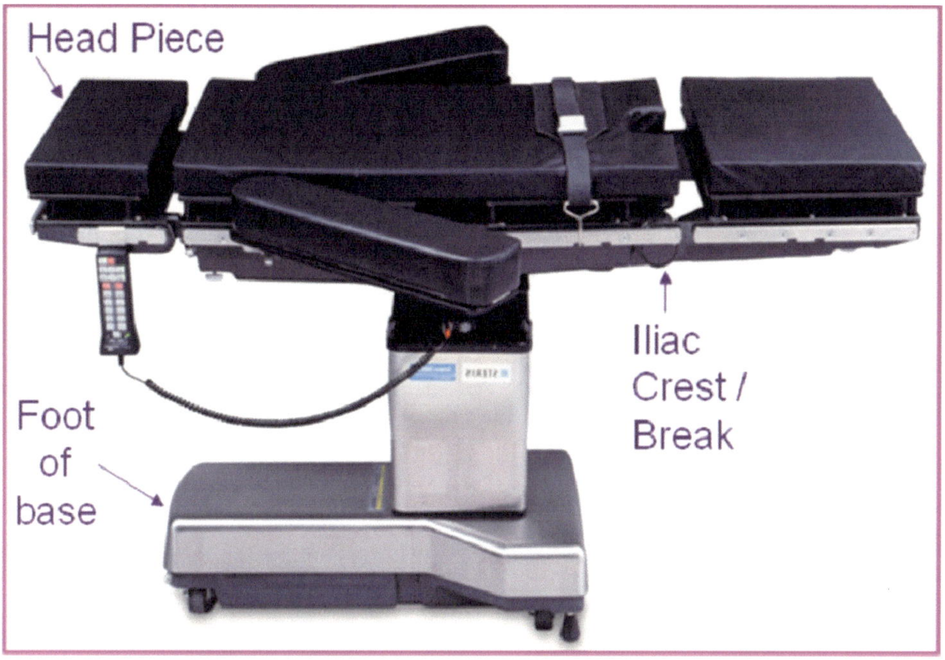

"Normal" table position: notice head piece over foot of base

Fig. 13. Standard orientation. To facilitate an successful lateral retroperitoneal transpsoas approach, the head piece must be switched.

Prior to positioning the patient, a left sided or right sided approach should be chosen considering the following factors.

- Previous unilateral retroperitoneal surgery.
- Position of iliac crest in relation to targeted disc space on pre operative plain films.
- Collapsed or open disc space, presence of lateral listhesis.
- In cases of degenerative scoliosis, convex or concave aspect of curve.
- Convenience of operating room set up.
- Vascular anomalies present on preoperative MRI that would preclude access.

In general, we typically chose a left sided access approach in most instances when all other variable have been accounted for to avoid vasculature and for convenience of OR setup.

The patient is then placed in the lateral position with an axillary roll and with all pressure points securely padded (Figure 14). The table should initially be flat and radiographs need to be obtained in a true lateral and AP plane during positioning prior to taping the patient into position.

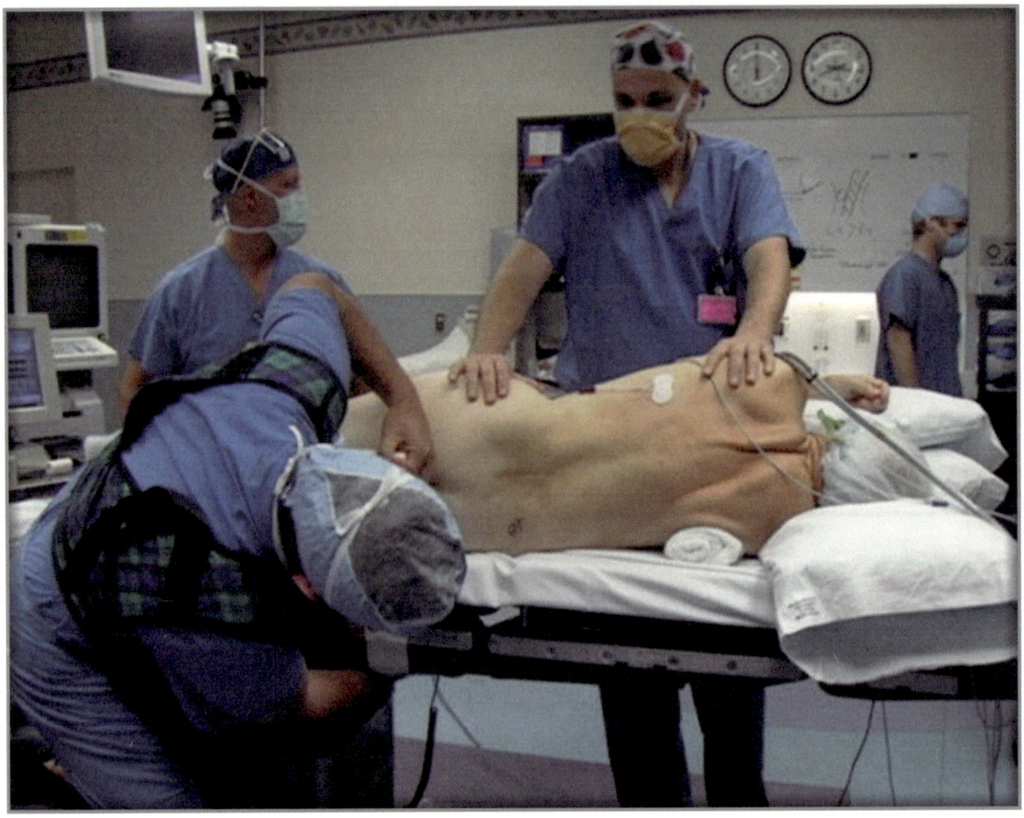

Fig. 14. Proper positioning of patient prior to taping and "breaking" table. The patient is then secure to the table at the following locations: just below the iliac crest (A), over the thoracic region (B), from the iliac crest to the knee, then to the table (C), from the table to the knee, past the ankle, then to the table (D) (Figure 15).

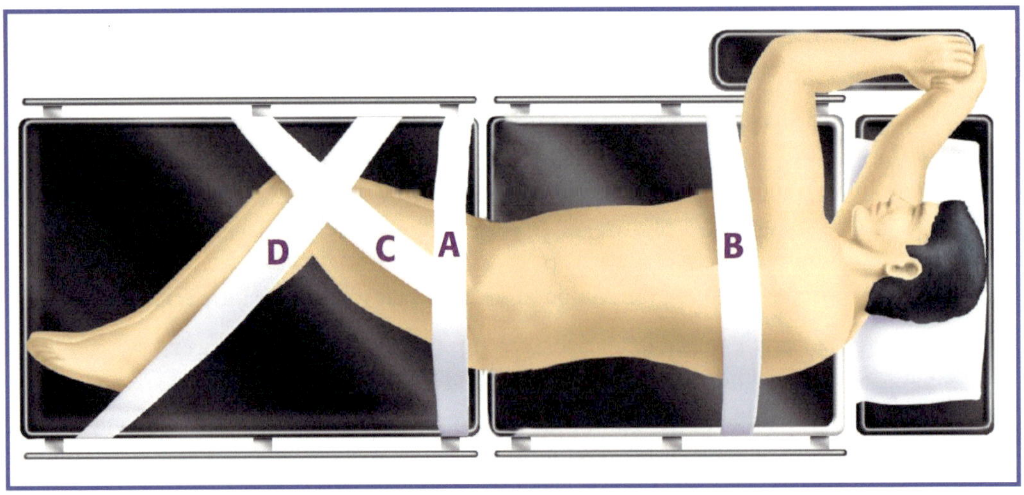

Fig. 15. Diagram showing correct placement of tape.

Next, the C-arm fluoroscopy unit is brought into the field and AP images are first obtained. In order to obtain the true images (Figure 16), the c-arm must match the lordotic angles of the spine. It is important at all times to maintain the fluoroscope at 90 degrees to the patient while rotating or tilting the table to obtain a true view. Indicators of a true AP image include midline spinous processes and symmetrical pedicles.

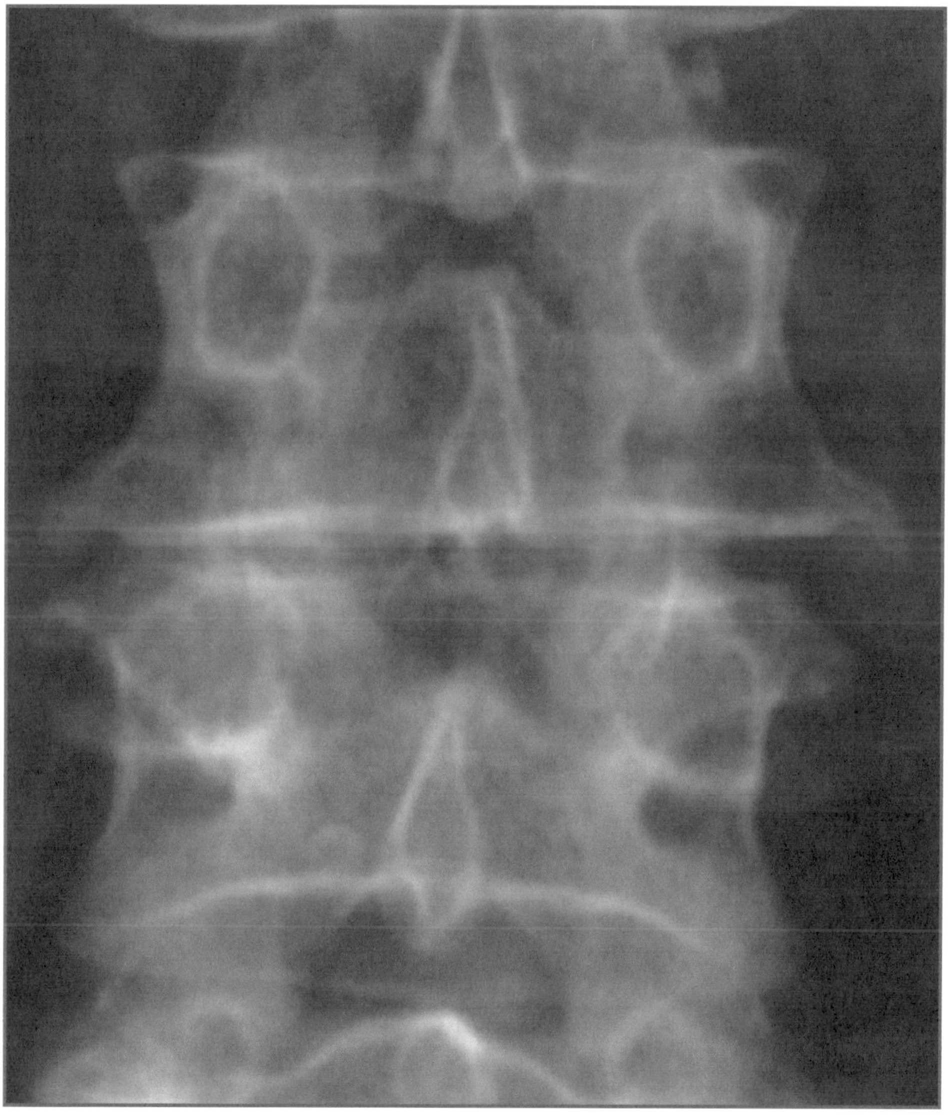

Fig. 16. True A/P image with spinous process centered and pedicles approximating their anatomic location at the endplate. Notice no "double endplate" shadow.

The table is flexed to open up the space between the rib cage and the iliac crest (Figure 17). Once again, patient positioning is crucial to success and ensuring the patient is positioned such that the spine will "open up" after the table is flexed is essential. The surgeon must work perpendicular to the floor and parallel to the disc space at all times to avoid inadvertent vascular or neural injury. Proper fluoroscopic aligment and meticulous attention to this principal will help avoid migration of instrumentation that may lead to vascular or neural injury.

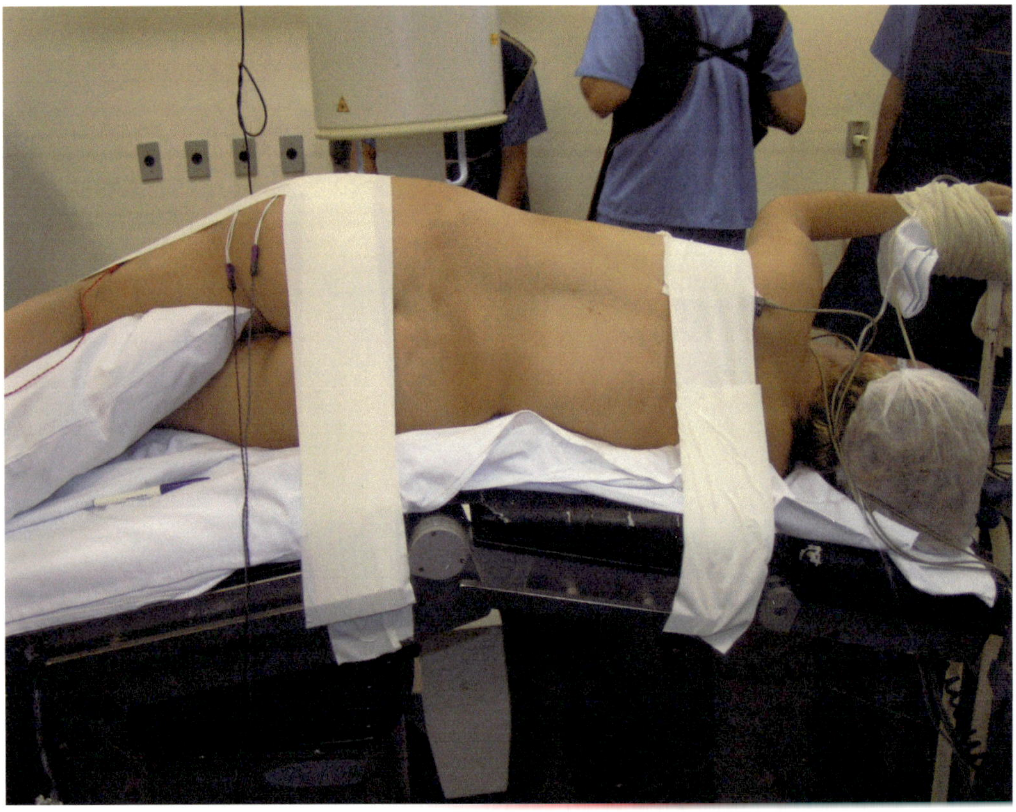

Fig. 17. Flexing the table after patient has been secured.

After an AP image has been obtained, the c-arm is rotated to obtain the lateral image. Once again, the c arm must be perpendicular to the floor. This helps to maintain a straight, up-down orientation and trajectory of all instruments being passed in and out of the disc. Failure to maintain a strict up-down orientation can result in serious vascular or neurologic injury caused by inappropriate trajectory. To obtain the true lateral image, the table can be adjusted in the "trendelenberg" fashion by reflexing the table head up. Indications of a true lateral projection include: linear endplates, linear posterior cortex, and superimposed pedicle (Figure 18).

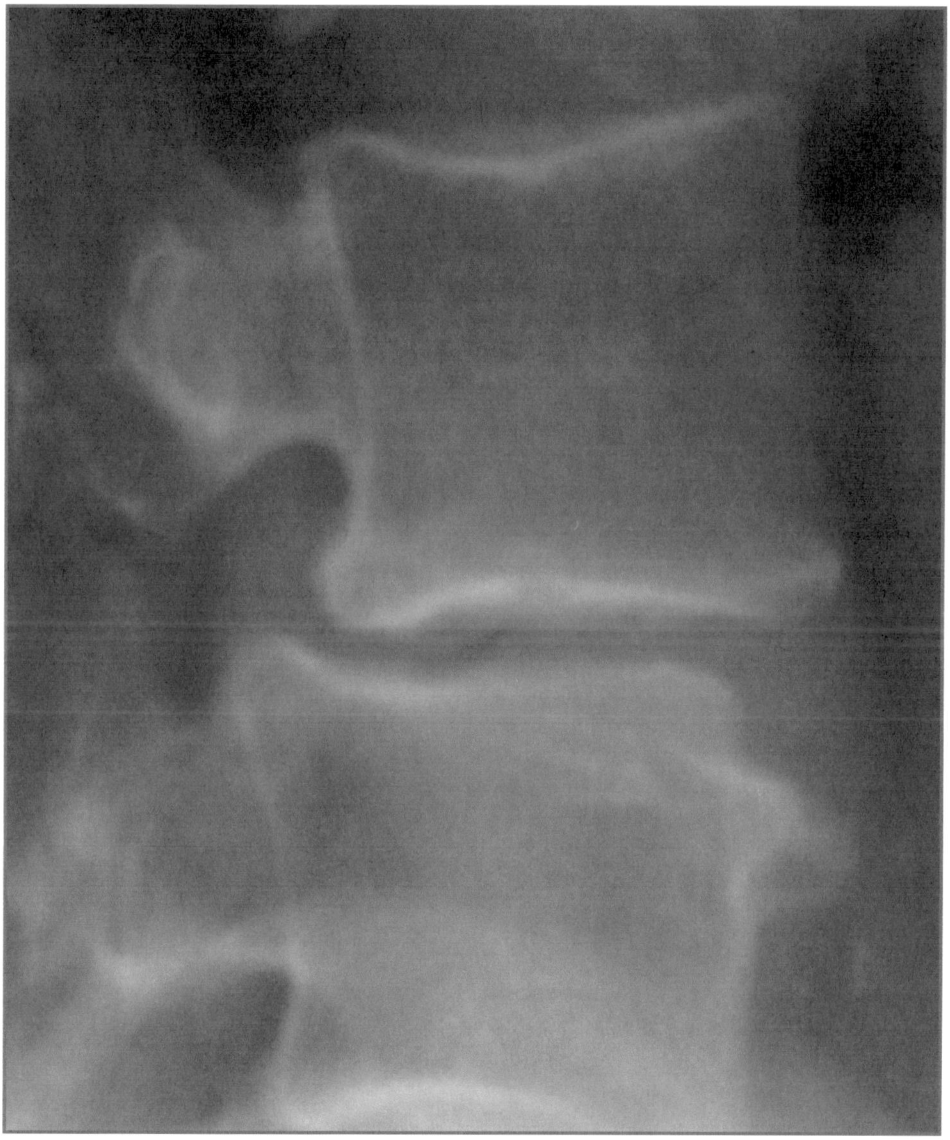

Fig. 18. True lateral image. Notice no "double pedicle" shadows. The disc space of interest is marked on AP and lateral views.

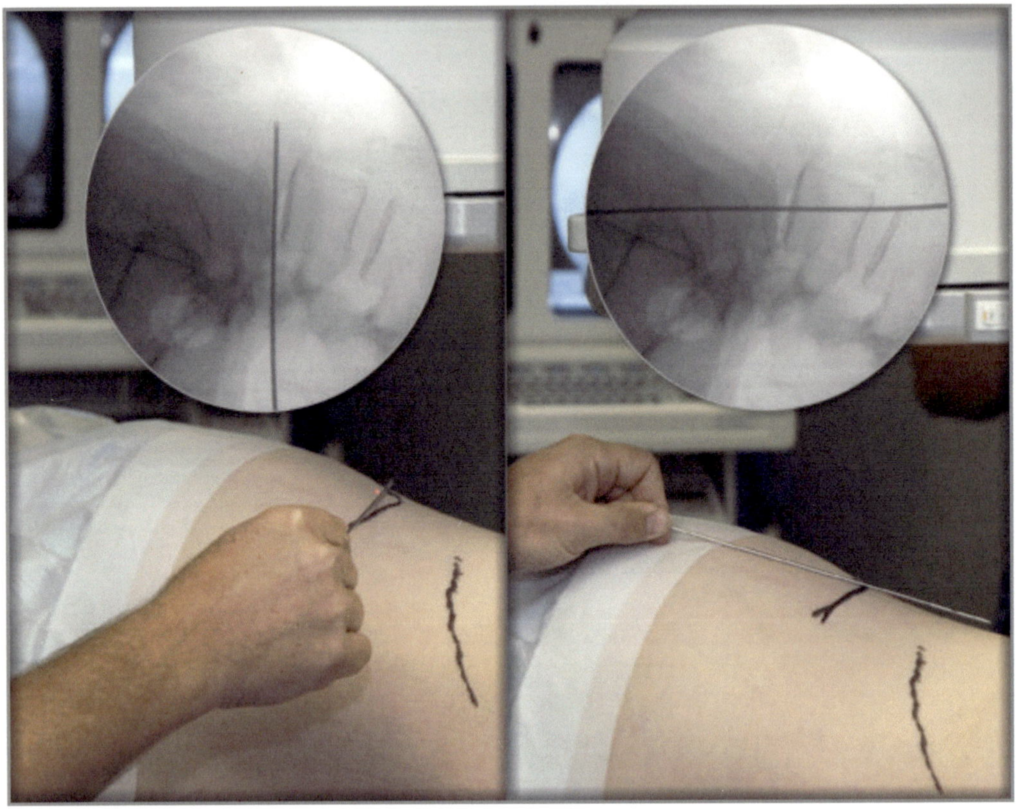

Fig. 19. Localizing the target prior to incision. Notice the first marker is marking the disc space and its orientation, and the second marker is located on the "safe zone" where the disc will be accessed.

After the patient is prepped and draped in the usual sterile fashion, one begins accessing the retroperitoneal space. The incision is based on the intersection of the K wires placed during AP and lateral localization(Figure 19). The mark is typically just lateral to the erector spinae muscles (Figure 20). An incision is made and through the posterolateral incision, the subcutaneous tissue layers are dissected using blunt scissors and findger dissection. After passing through the abdominal musculature; using a loss of resistance to guage depth results in an indication that the retroperitoneal space has been reached. A finger is passed into the retroperitoneal space and in a gentle sweeping motion is used to ensure that the peritoneum is released anteriorly, and to ensure that the abdominal contents have been mobilized forward. At our institution, we typically use a single incision and work through a incision between the intermusclular septum just lateral to the junction of the erector spinae musculature, the quadrates lumborum and the psoas.

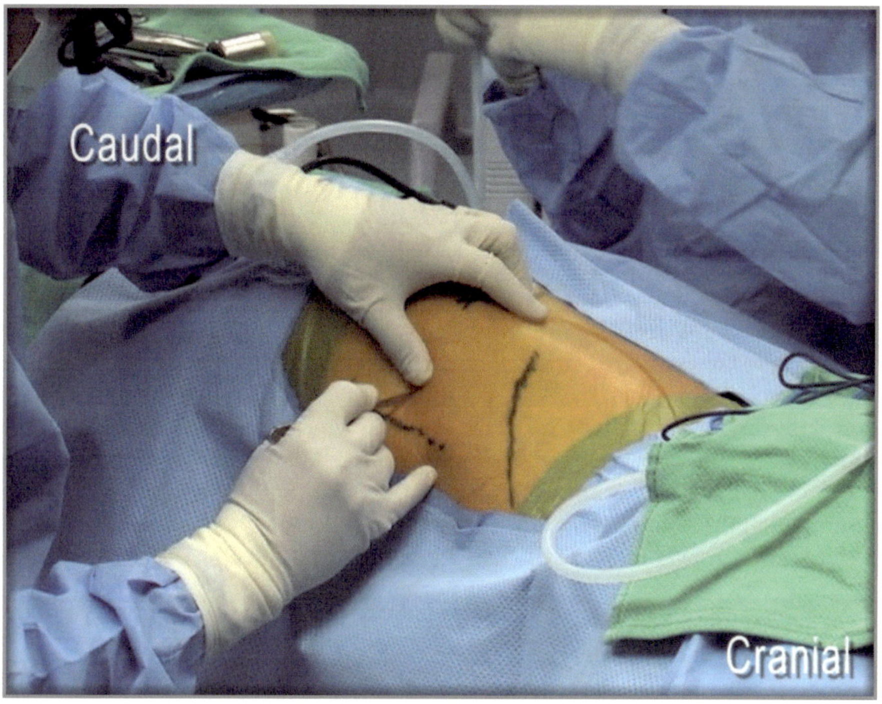

Fig. 20. The incision is made just lateral the erector spinae muscles.

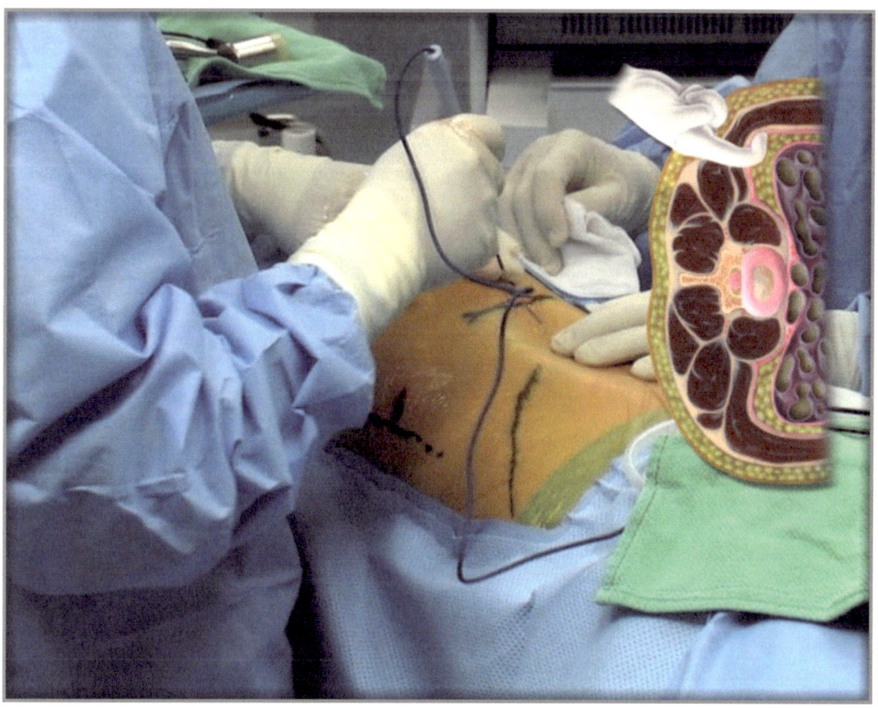

Fig. 21. Locating the point through which the dilators will be passed.

When the peritoneal space is encountered , the surgeon palpates for the psoas muscle using the anterior tip of the transverse process as a landmark for identification. After locating the psoas muscle, the index finger is passed under the abdominal wall to lie directly underneath the lateral skin mark ensuring the abdominal contents are free from passage of the dilators. A second incision is made at this point through which the initial dilator will be passed(Figure 21). The first of sequential dilators is then connect to the neuromonioring system and then passed through the incision to inside the retroperitoneal space where the index finger will guide it onto the psoas muscle.

Once the initial dilator contacts the psoas muscle, and image is obtained using the intraopeartive c-arm fluoroscopy unit in the lateral position(Figure 22). The ideal location for the intial dilator on imaging is the center (or just posterior to the center) of the disc space. With the neuromonitoring unit in place, the fibers of the psoas muscle are split using blunt dissection with the initial dilator. The dilator is slowly advanced through the psoas in the Detection mode to identify and avoid nerves of the lumbosacral plexus. If the dilator approaches a nerve, it is slowly rotated 360 degrees to determine the location of the nerve. A higher stimulation threshold indicates that the nerve is on the distal side of the tip. In which case, the dilator is removed, then reoriented and a new path through the psoas is taken.

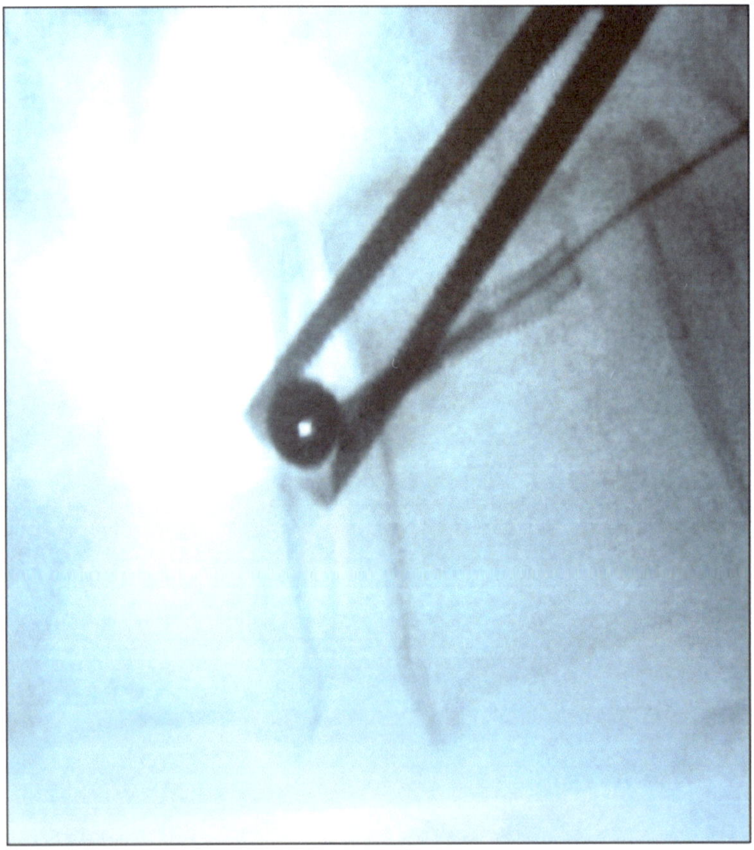

Fig. 22. The initial dilator is seen resting on the surface of the psoas muscle and appears to be in a safe location.

The retractor is then assembled with the appropriate length blades and inserted over the dilators. The retractor can also be connected to the neuromonitoring system and stimulated as it is inserted (Figure 23). Once inserted, initial retractor depth can be confirmed with imaging. Two attachment points allow migration of the blades. A center attachment ensures that the blades open only anterior to that position, and attachment to the posterior point of connection ensure that the blades open only posterior. Care must be taken to ensure then plades don't compress neural elements against the transverse process. Illumination is achieved via the light cables down the blades of the retractor.

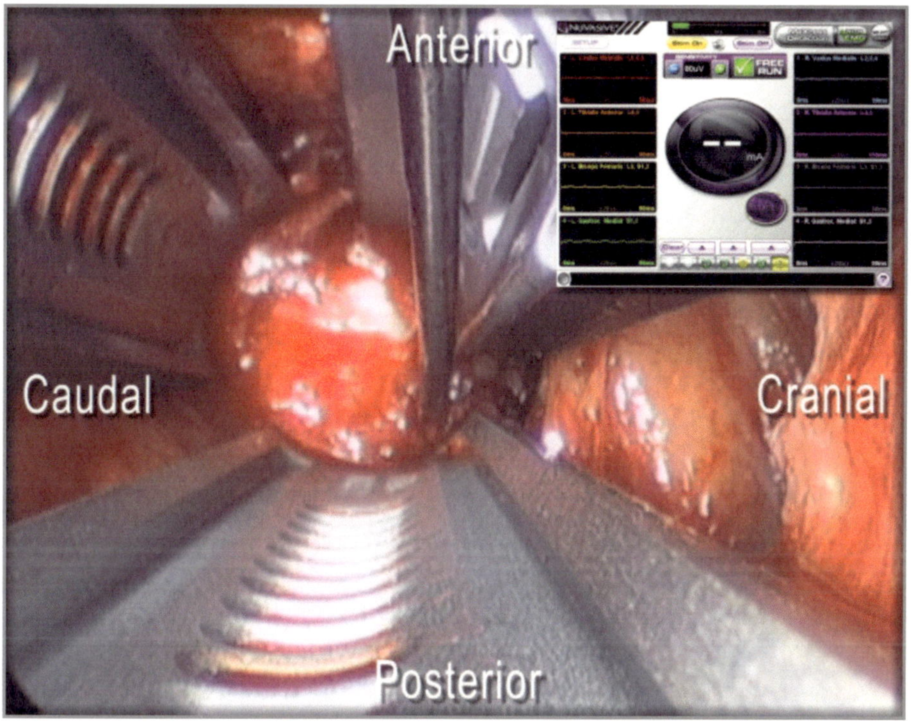

Fig. 23. View through the retractor system after passing through the posas muscle.

The neuromonitoring probe is then used to palpate the field exposed by the retractors to ensure no neural elements are within the operative field. Distal exposure can be achieved by using the blade rotation wrenches to gain optimal access to the disc space. At this point, fixation shims can be added to the retractor construct for additional stabilization. Addition of a stabilizing shim is recommended in revision surgeries, presence of a high riding crest at L4/5, or ribs at L1/2. Before placement of shims, one must identify where it will engage, visually check the area for nerves and segmental vessels, and test for nerves with the neuromonitoring probe.

2.5 Discectomy

Once the operative corridor has been established, the disc space can be prepared. After performing an annulotomy (at least 18mm to accommodate implant), the disc space can be prepared using a combination of Rongeurs, Currettes, and Rasps. Contralateral annular release is imperative to the procedure to achieve proper coronal alignment. The can be safely performed by passing a Cobb elevator along both superior and inferior endplates completely through the contralateral annulus (Figures 24-25). This allows placement of an implant on the ring apophysis bilaterally.

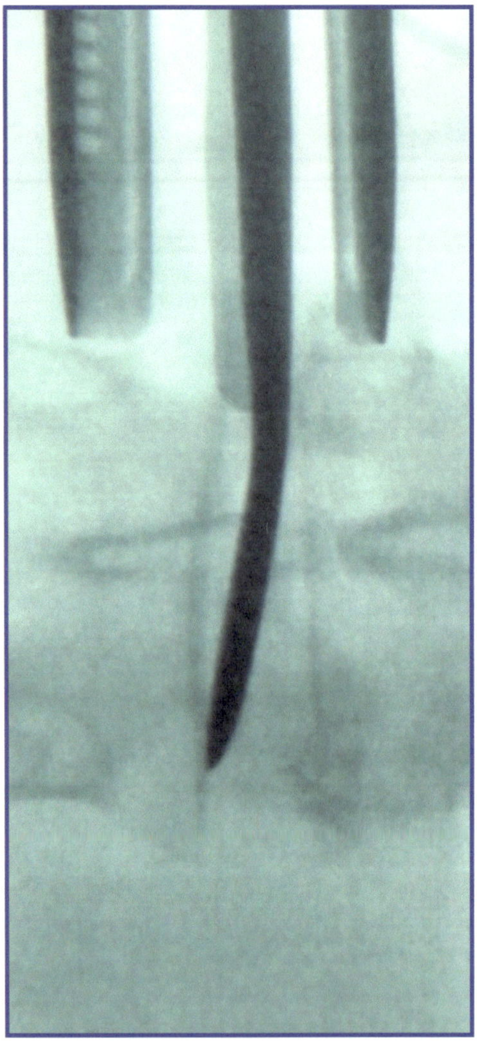

Fig. 24. Preparation of the disc space with Cobb elevator.

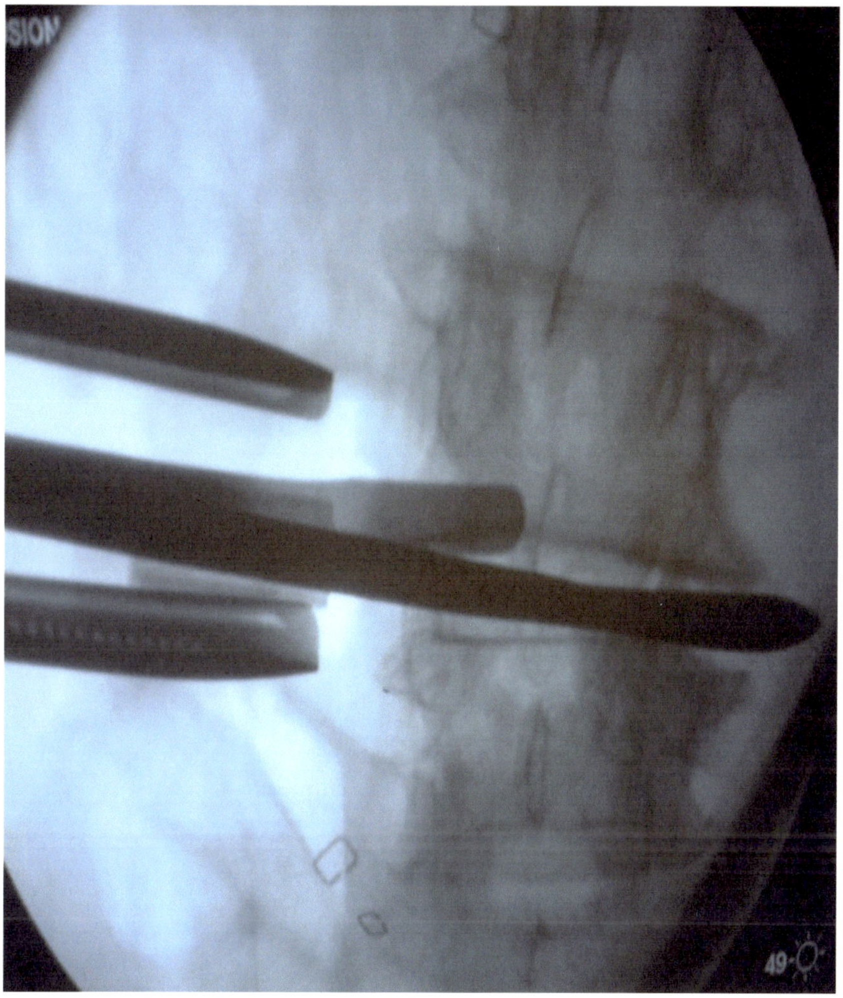

Fig. 25. Contralateral annular release with Cobb elevator. This is crucial for appropriate graft placement and restoration of coronal balance.

2.6 Grafting

After the discectomy has been performed and the endplates have been prepared, the next step is to choose an appropriately sized implant. A benefit of the lateral approach is the ability to place a large implant that engages the densest areas of endplate support (Figures 26-27). The implant length should thus span the ring apophysis and align with the lateral borders of the endplates on an AP image. The height of the implant should be chosen on basis of adequate disc height restoration without placing excessive s train on the anterior longitudinal ligament or the endplates. Reappoximation of saggital alignment can be achieved by choosing a lordotic graft or via a more central to anterior placement of the implant. Restoration of disc height also indirectly decompresses the foramen and centrally via corrections in disc height, sagittal and coronal alignment and anterior and lateral listhesis.

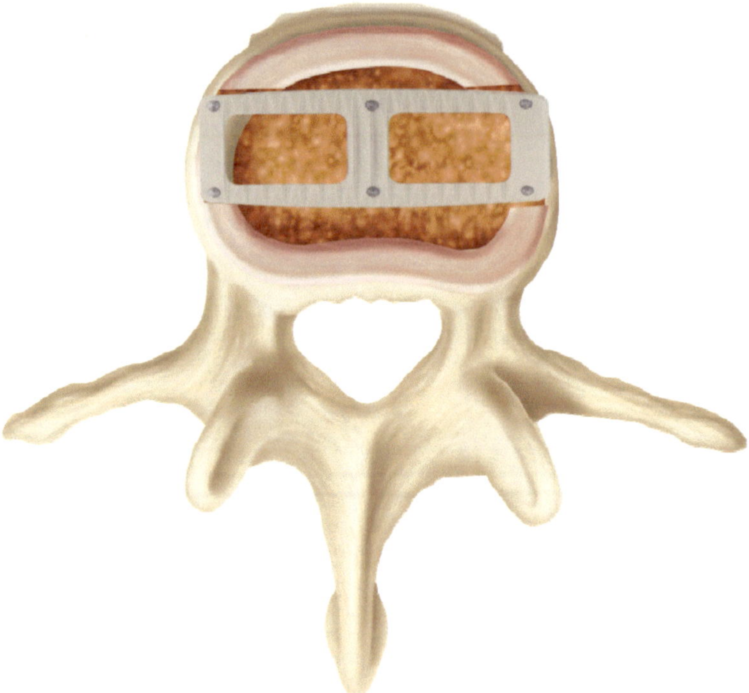

Fig. 26. Artists illustration of placement of graft demonstrating wide footprint and spanning the ring apophysis and areas of maximum structural support.

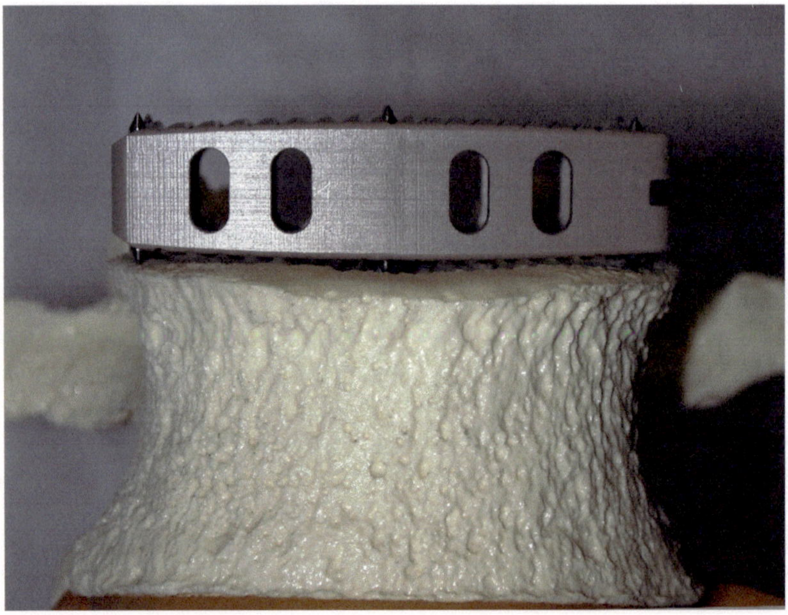

Fig. 27. A/P view of interbody graft on model shows graft spanning the areas of densest cortical bone.

The distractor and dilators are used to gauge the appropriate sized trial which is then impacted into the disc space under fluoroscopic guidance. Once an appropriate sized trial is placed, its position is verified with AP and lateral fluoroscopy. An implant is chosen, then filled with graft material and or a biological adjuvant (rh-BMP, Medronic Sofamor-Danek, Memphis, TN). The implant is then impacted into the disc space under AP fluoroscopy. Once a trial has been placed, its location is confirmed under AP and lateral fluoroscopy prior to positioning the implant. The ideal position is centered across the disc space from a medial-lateral perspective, and in the anterior to medial third of the disc space from an anterior to posterior perspective (Figure 28).

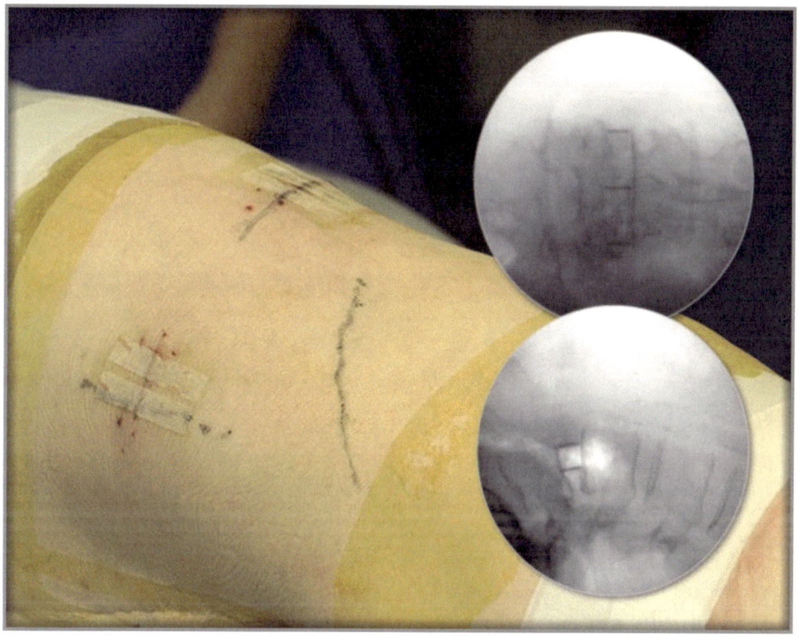

Fig. 28. A/P and lateral radiographs showing ideal graft positioning at conclusion of procedure.

2.7 Closing/postoperative

After conclusion of the procedure, the bladed retractors are removed and the soft tissues are inspected for any bleeding in the posas muscle or disc space. The wound is closed in layers paying meticulous attention to detailed wound closure. It is helpful to reflex the bed to a more anatomically correct position to facilitate wound closure in a tensionless fashion. Supplemental posterior instrumentation is added as needed.

Postoperative pain for the lateral incision tends to be minimial, however there are some transient side effects to expect, and these should be discussed with the patient during the preoperative office visits. Tenderness with hip flexion on the operative side is common and resolves spontaneously. Eight to 10% of patients experience some initial psoas weakness which typically resolves within 1-2 weeks. Seven transpsoas outcome studies have described sensory abnormalities in 0-30% of patients immediately after surgery. Complete resolution typically occurs by a year. From our own series, 50% of patients with new sensory abnormalities recover within 90 days, and nearly all within a year. There were low rates of patients who continued to report thigh numbness (7%) and pain (5.5%) beyond one year. Meticulous surgical technique and use of intraoperative monitoring can help avoid some complications. In general we avoid poor patient position, excessive passes of the intial dilator ("wanding") through the posas, and avoiding monopolar electrocautery. We encourage early ambularion, and use neurontin or imipramine for painful postoperative dysesthesias.

2.8 Case considerations

The patient is a 46 year old active male with axial low back pain, no leg pain, and no prior history of surgery. Physical examination revealed normal motor strength with no functional deficits. Femoral and straight leg testing did not produce radicular pain.

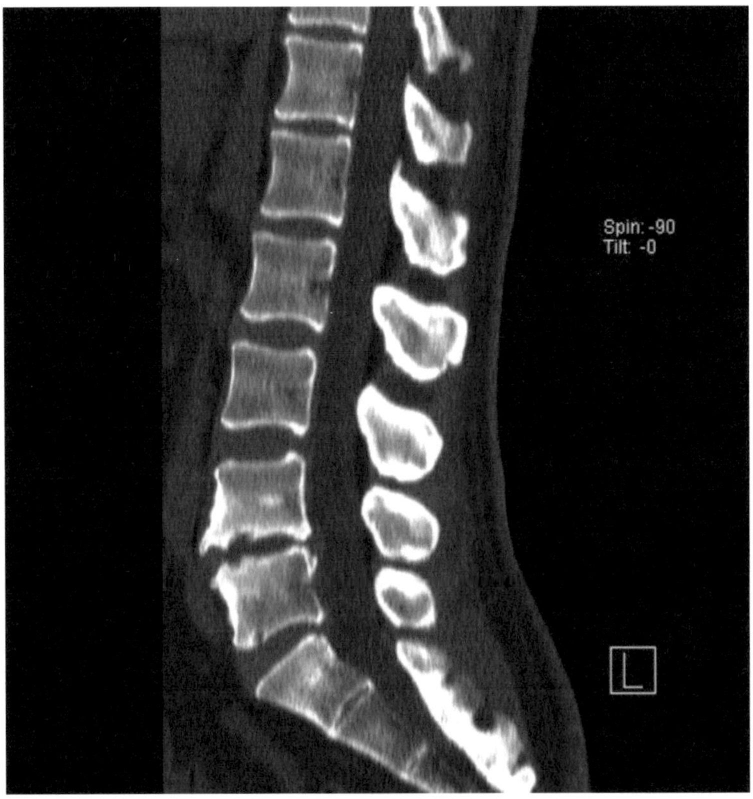

Fig. 29. CT of lumbar spine with saggital reconstruction showing advanced disc degeneration.

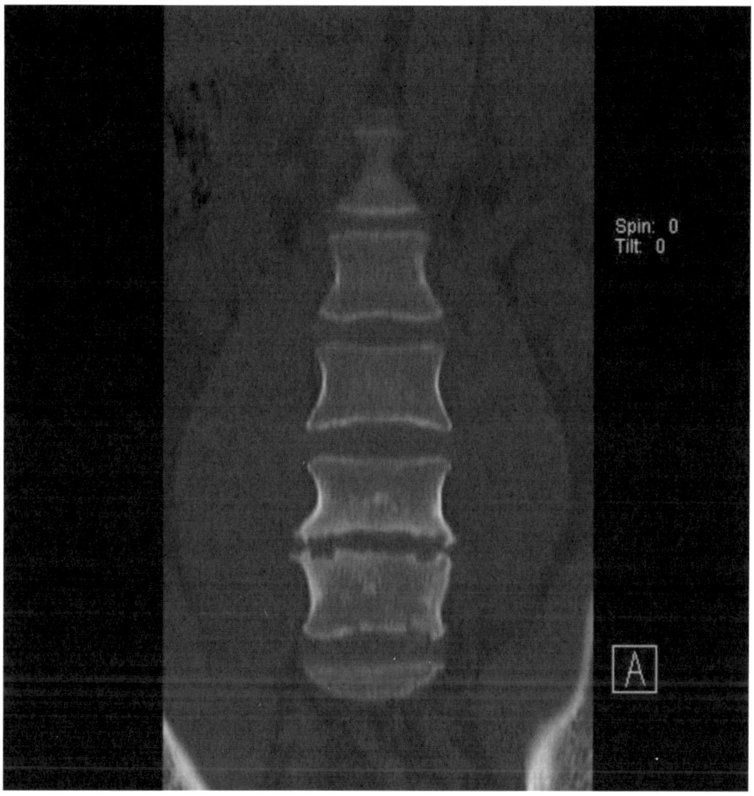

Fig. 30. CT of lumbar spine with coronal reconstruction showing advanced disc degeneration.

CT of the lumbar spine with saggital reconstruction demonstrated endplate changes consistent with sclerotic adaptations of advanced disc degeneration (Figures 29-30). MRI (not shown) showed loss of T2 signal intensity in the disc space, no significant protrusions or annular tears, but a broad based collapse of the posterior annulus toward the canal.

Surgical options were discussed with the patient after he had failed an adequate trial of conservative management. The use of spinal fusion for DDD has be found to beneficial for many patients[18]. However, even with a successful posterior fusion, a number of patients contine to have pain from micromotion of the collapsed disc. The addition of an interbody graft increases the stability of the construct and can be performed via a midline posterior approach as a PLIF or TLIF, or anterior via and ALIF. The surgical goal was stabilization of the affected level, to restore height and to avoid over distraction of the facets. We offered the patient a lateral interbody fusion.

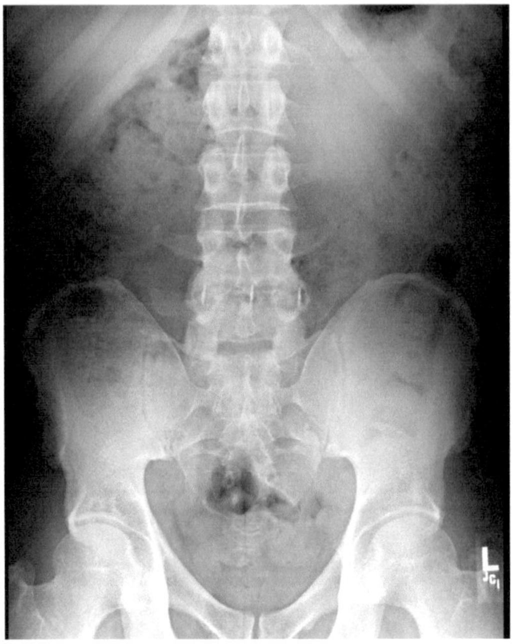

Fig. 31. Post operative A/P radiograph showing stand alone lateral interbody fusion. Note the preservation of coronal balance and restoration of disc space height.

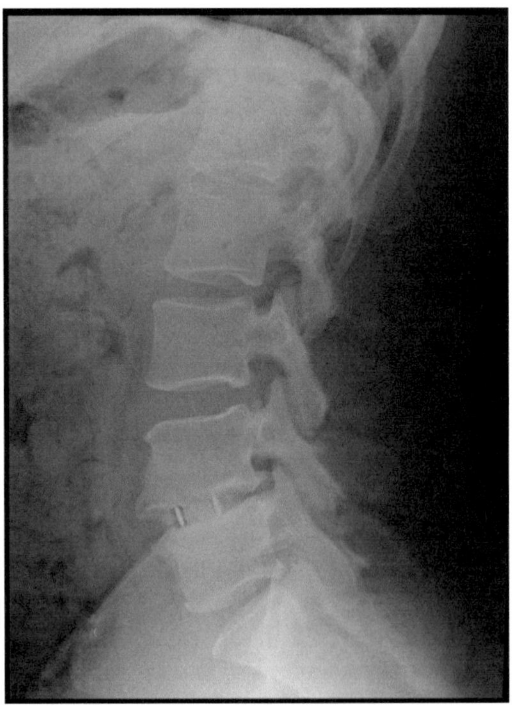

Fig. 32. Post operative lateral radiograph of stand alone lateral interbody fusion. Notice the preservation of lordosis, restoration of foramenal volume and disc space height.

Case one:

An 18 year old female fell from a two story roof and presented to the emergency room with ASIA C quadriplegia from an L2 burst fracture(Figures 33-34).

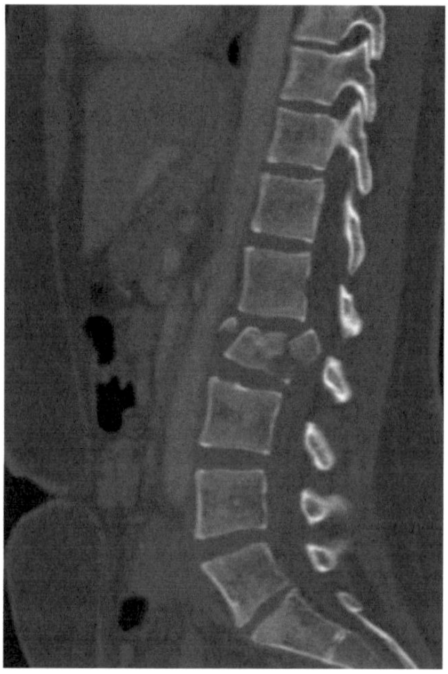

Fig. 33. CT of lumbar spine with saggital reconstruction showing L2 burst fracture with retropulsed fragments.

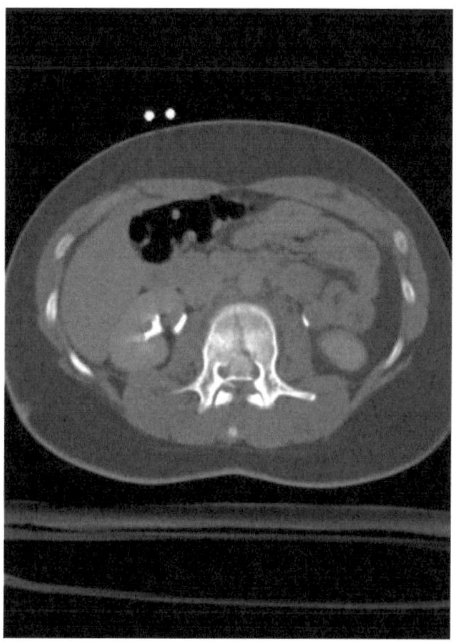

Fig. 34. Axial CT scan through L2 burst fracture showing retropulsed fragments and fractured vertebral body.

The patient underwent a L2 corpectomy via an XLIF approach and was fitted with an expandable titanium cage. The construct was supplemented by percutaneous pedicle screw fixation (Figures 35-38).

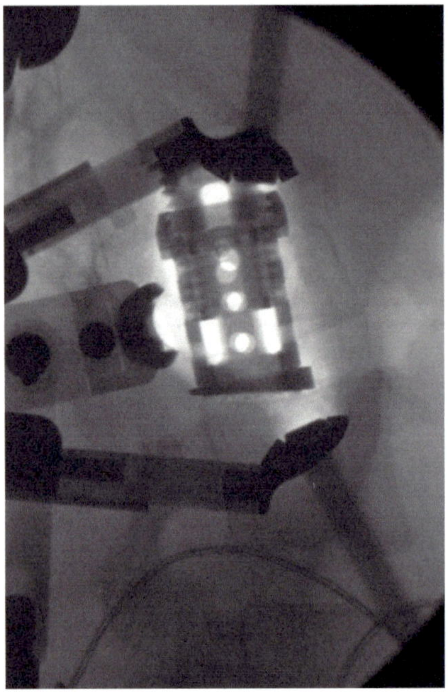

Fig. 35. Intraopeartive lateral C arm fluoroscopic image of expandable cage being deployed. Notice the adequate space provided by via a minimally invasive approach.

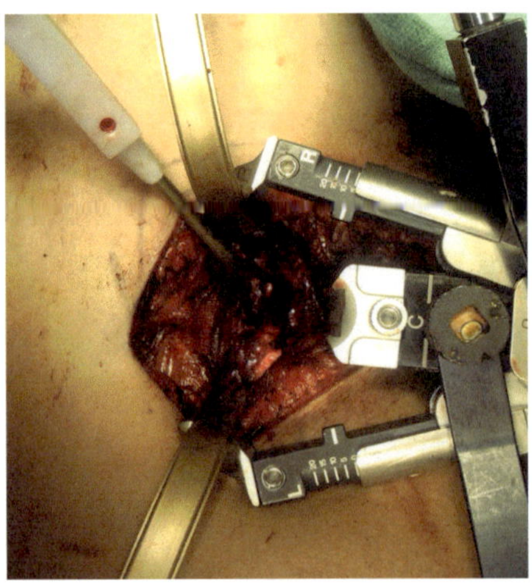

Fig. 36. View of the incision and position of the retractor system.

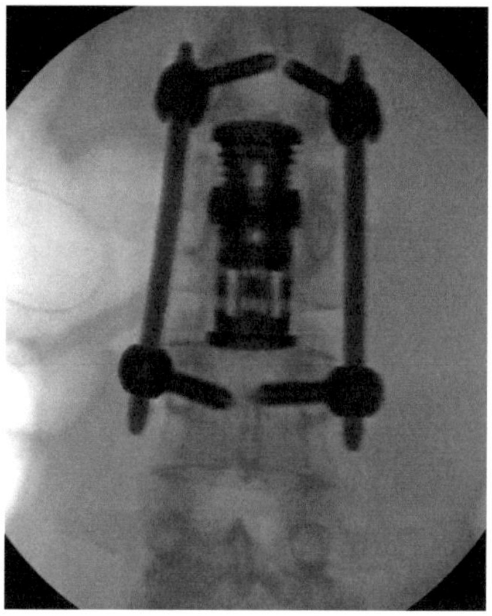

Fig. 37. Post operative A/P flurouscopic image of expandable cage and percutaneous pedicle screws.

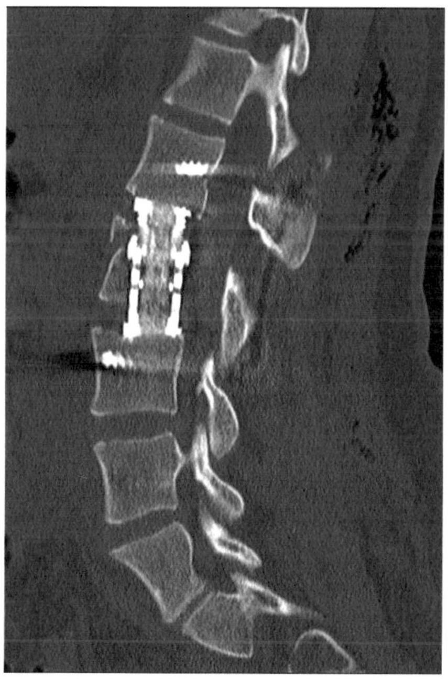

Fig. 38. Post operative CT of lumbar spine with saggital reconstruction showing complete decompression of canal via a lateral retroperitoneal transpsoas approach.

When performing corpectomies for trauma the surgical goal is immediate decompression which is often hampered by the need for an access surgeon. With the XLIF approach, this is eliminated. Additionally, in anterior approaches there is concern about posterior migration of fragments injuring the neural elements. By using an XLIF approach, and working within the retractors that border the adjacent vertebral segments as well as the thecal sac, the risk of posterior fragment migration is decreased. The XLIF approach allows decompression of the neural elements as well as restoration of anterior column support, is safe and reproducible.

Case two:

A 79 year old female presented with intractable back pain. She gives a history of having a spinal epidural abscess three years prior that was treated with multi-level laminectomies. She is currently neurologically intact, but requires a walker to stand up straight (Figures 39-42).

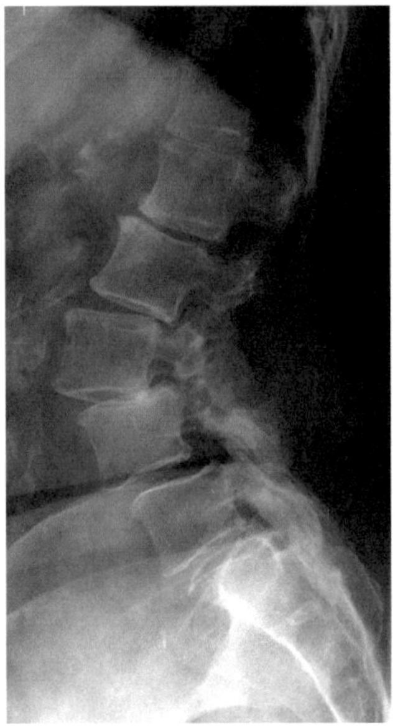

Fig. 39. Lateral plain radiograph demonstrating post-laminectomy deformity.

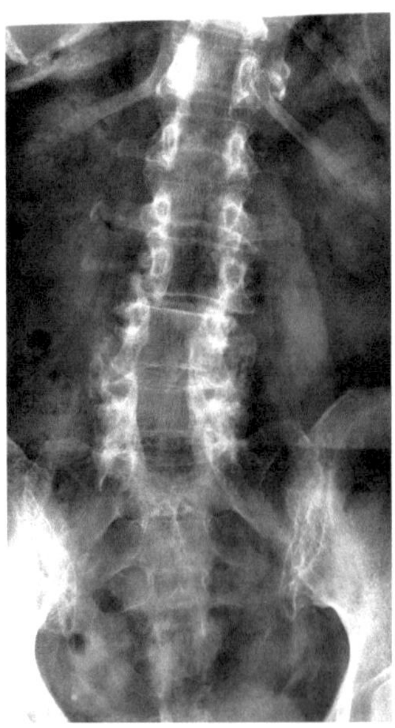

Fig. 40. A/P radiograph demonstrating coronal deformity in addition to saggital deformity.

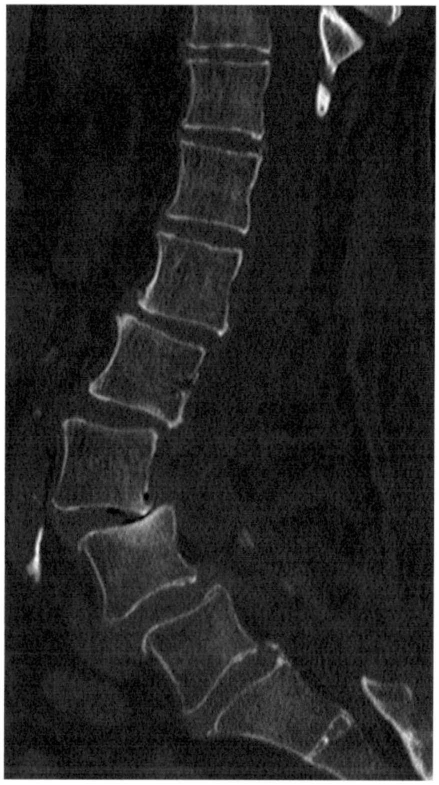

Fig. 41. CT of lumbar spine with saggital reconstruction demonstrating the degree of post-laminectomy deformity.

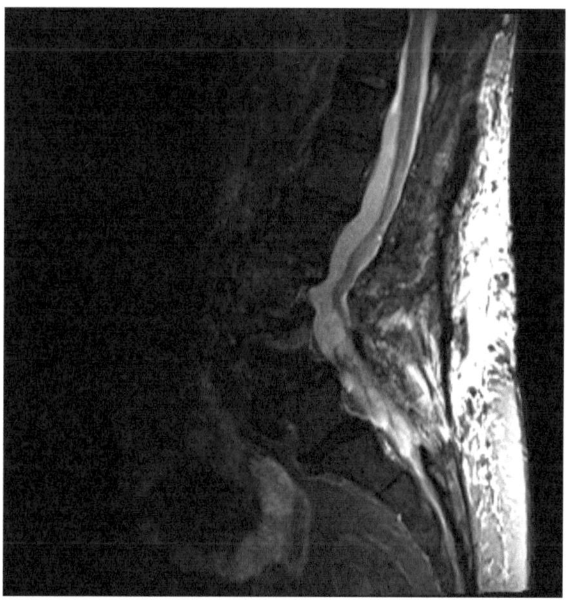

Fig. 42. Saggital T2 weighted MRI of same patient.

Traditional treatments for iatrogenic deformity are associated with long operative times, high blood loss, and extended hospitalization. As surgical magnitude increae, morbidity, complication and recovery times increase substantially. The lateral retroperitoneal transposas approach results in minimal dissection and stripping result in less surgical time and less bleeding. The bilateral annular relase allows straightening and derotation of the spine. Placing large interbody implants realigns the endplates, restores disc heights and indirectly decompresses the neural elements. Saggital balance can be restored through the placement of lordotic grafts in the anterior disc space (Figures 43-44). The lateral retroperitoneal transposas approach offers a more tolerable surgical option for patients with complex deformity and significant medical comorbidities.

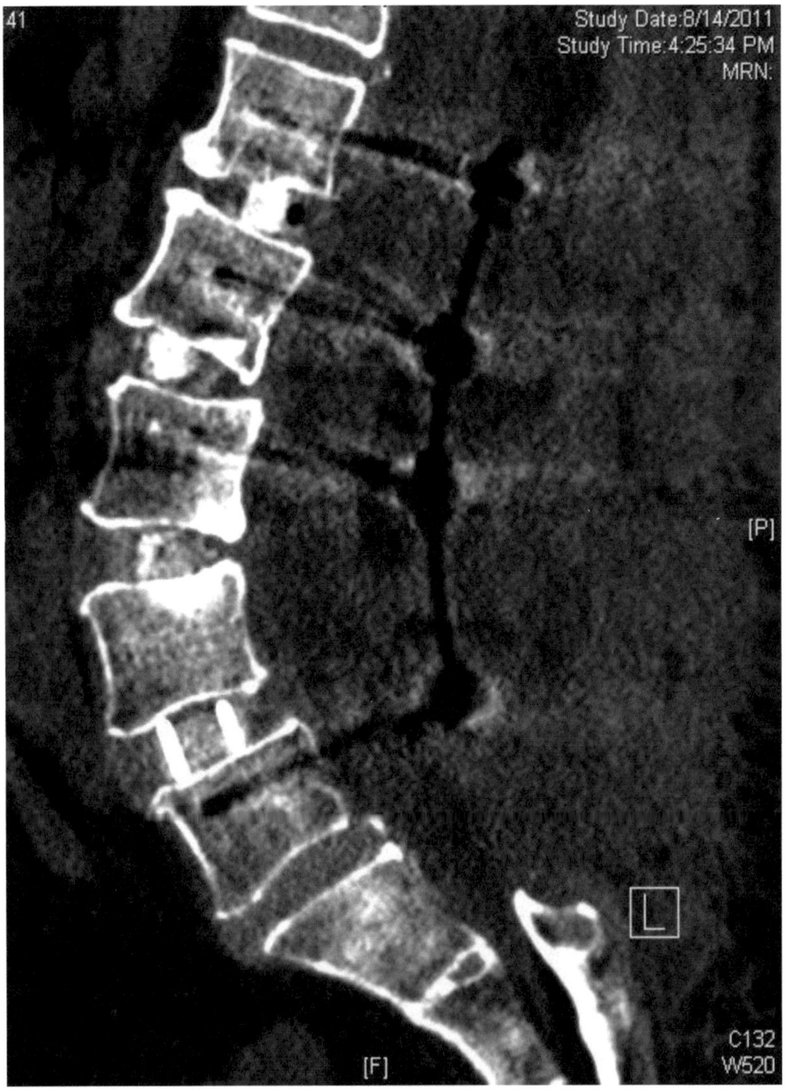

Fig. 43. Post operative CT of lumbar spine with saggital reconstruction demonstrating restoration of saggital balance.

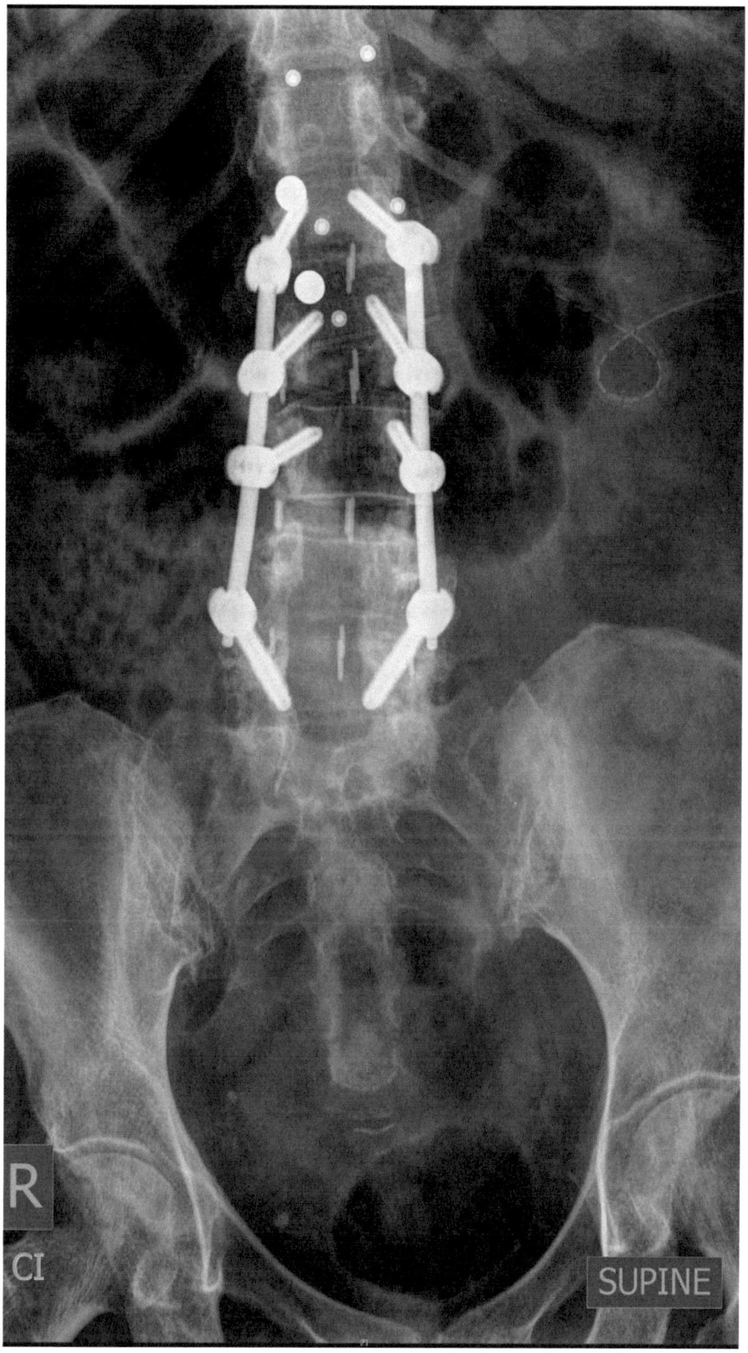

Fig. 44. Post operative A/P radiograph demonstrating restoration of coronal balance.

3. Acknowledgment

The authors would like to thank NuVasive (San Diego, CA) for figures 1-8, 13-15, 17, 19-28.

4. References

[1] Burns B. An Operation for Spondylolisthesis. *Lancet.* 1933 1933;1(23):33.

[2] Bohm H, Harms J, Donk R, Zielke K. Correction and stabilization of angular kyphosis. *Clin Orthop Relat Res.* Sep 1990(258):56-61.

[3] Bradford DS. Adult scoliosis. Current concepts of treatment. *Clin Orthop Relat Res.* Apr 1988(229):70-87.

[4] Gertzbein SD, Court-Brown CM, Jacobs RR, et al. Decompression and circumferential stabilization of unstable spinal fractures. *Spine (Phila Pa 1976).* Aug 1988;13(8):892-895.

[5] Cloward RB. The treatment of ruptured lumbar intervertebral discs by vertebral body fusion. I. Indications, operative technique, after care. *J Neurosurg.* Mar 1953;10(2):154-168.

[6] Faciszewski T, Winter RB, Lonstein JE, Denis F, Johnson L. The surgical and medical perioperative complications of anterior spinal fusion surgery in the thoracic and lumbar spine in adults. A review of 1223 procedures. *Spine (Phila Pa 1976).* Jul 15 1995;20(14):1592-1599.

[7] Regan JJ, Aronoff RJ, Ohnmeiss DD, Sengupta DK. Laparoscopic approach to L4-L5 for interbody fusion using BAK cages: experience in the first 58 cases. *Spine (Phila Pa 1976).* Oct 15 1999;24(20):2171-2174.

[8] Baker JK, Reardon PR, Reardon MJ, Heggeness MH. Vascular injury in anterior lumbar surgery. *Spine (Phila Pa 1976).* Nov 1993;18(15):2227-2230.

[9] Christensen FB, Bunger CE. Retrograde ejaculation after retroperitoneal lower lumbar interbody fusion. *Int Orthop.* 1997;21(3):176-180.

[10] Hackenberg L, Liljenqvist U, Halm H, Winkelmann W. Occlusion of the left common iliac artery and consecutive thromboembolism of the left popliteal artery following anterior lumbar interbody fusion. *J Spinal Disord.* Aug 2001;14(4):365-368.

[11] Hannon JK, Faircloth WB, Lane DR, et al. Comparison of insufflation vs. retractional technique for laparoscopic-assisted intervertebral fusion of the lumbar spine. *Surg Endosc.* Mar 2000;14(3):300-304.

[12] McAfee PC, Bohlman HH, Yuan HA. Anterior decompression of traumatic thoracolumbar fractures with incomplete neurological deficit using a retroperitoneal approach. *J Bone Joint Surg Am.* Jan 1985;67(1):89-104.

[13] Mayer HM. A new microsurgical technique for minimally invasive anterior lumbar interbody fusion. *Spine (Phila Pa 1976).* Mar 15 1997;22(6):691-699; discussion 700.

[14] McAfee PC, Regan JJ, Geis WP, Fedder IL. Minimally invasive anterior retroperitoneal approach to the lumbar spine. Emphasis on the lateral BAK. *Spine (Phila Pa 1976).* Jul 1 1998;23(13):1476-1484.

[15] Bergey DL, Villavicencio AT, Goldstein T, Regan JJ. Endoscopic lateral transpsoas approach to the lumbar spine. *Spine (Phila Pa 1976).* Aug 1 2004;29(15):1681-1688.

[16] Ozgur BM, Aryan HE, Pimenta L, Taylor WR. Extreme Lateral Interbody Fusion (XLIF): a novel surgical technique for anterior lumbar interbody fusion. *Spine J.* Jul-Aug 2006;6(4):435-443.

[17] White AA, Panjabi MM. *Clinical biomechanics of the spine.* 2nd ed. Philadelphia: Lippincott; 1990.

[18] Nachemson A, Zdeblick TA, O'Brien JP. Lumbar disc disease with discogenic pain. What surgical treatment is most effective? *Spine (Phila Pa 1976).* Aug 1 1996;21(15):1835-1838.

6

The Minimally Invasive Retroperitoneal Transpsoas Approach

Tien V. Le and Juan S. Uribe
Department of Neurosurgery and Brain Repair, University of South Florida, Tampa, Florida, USA

1. Introduction

Minimally invasive spine surgery has evolved from traditional open spine surgery, and it is an accepted, safe alternative (McAfee, et al., 2010). Traditional open operations for lumbar interbody fusion include anterior lumbar interbody fusion (ALIF), posterior lumbar interbody fusion (PLIF), and transforaminal lumbar interbody fusion (TLIF). The ALIF provides for a large interbody graft for disc space re-expansion, restoration of lumbar lordosis, and elimination of discogenic pain (Hodgson & Stock, 1956). In addition, posterior facet joint complexes and tension bands remain intact. However, an access surgeon may be needed, and complications can include a risk of vascular injury and also rare iatrogenic retrograde ejaculation in males postoperatively. The TLIF (Harms & Rolinger, 1982; Harms & Jeszenszky, 1998) was developed as a modification of the PLIF (Cloward, 1953) to decrease the degree of nerve root and thecal sac manipulation, and it allows for interbody fusion, concurrent posterior segmental instrumentation, and circumferential fusion. It can be performed either in an open or minimally invasive manner. The graft size is typically smaller than that of the ALIF, however.

First introduced by Luiz Pimenta in 2001, the retroperitoneal transpsoas minimally invasive lateral interbody fusion (MIS LIF) is a safe and effective alternative to anterior or posterior approaches for lumbar fusion (Pimenta, 2001; Ozgur, et al., 2006). Advantages include indirect neurological decompression with less tissue trauma, minimal blood loss, shorter operation times, less wound issues, placement of a larger cage, and early patient mobilization (Eck, et al., 2007; Benglis, et al., 2008; Wang, et al., 2008; Uribe, et al., 2010). In addition, normal stabilizing ligaments are not sacrificed as compared to other interbody techniques.

This technique was an adaptation of an endoscopic lateral transpsoas approach to lumbar fusion as described by Bergey et al. (Bergey, et al., 2004). They found that the endoscopic lateral transpsoas approach to the lumbar spine was a safe method to fuse the lumbar vertebrae, which allowed for exposure of the lumbar spine without mobilization of the great vessels or sympathetic plexus.

Today, there are several systems from various manufacturers that will allow for an MIS lateral retroperitoneal transpsoas approach. The two most common are the eXtreme Lateral Interbody Fusion/XLIF® (NuVasive, San Diego, CA) and Direct Lateral Interbody Fusion/DLIF® (Medtronic, Memphis, TN).

Clinical applications of the retroperitoneal transpsoas MIS LIF include a wide range of spinal conditions including trauma, adult degenerative scoliosis, degenerative disc disease, spondylosis with instability, lumbar stenosis, spondylolisthesis, tumor, and adjacent segment failure. Research on MIS LIF is very active, and clinical outcomes appear to be promising.

2. Anatomic considerations

The lateral approach may be unfamiliar to spine surgeons who are accustomed to a posterior approach. Because of this, a review of key anatomic structures encountered with the lateral approach is paramount. In the order encountered, the muscles include the external oblique, internal oblique, and the transversus abdominis muscle. Once the retroperitoneal space is entered, the quadratus lumborum and psoas muscle are then encountered. The details of blunt dissection, as opposed to electrocautery, are discussed later, but careful attention must be paid in order to avoid injuring a traversing lumbar plexus nerve, which could lead to postoperative deficits.

2.1 The lumbar plexus

The lumbar plexus is found within the substance of the psoas muscle. It is a part of the lumbosacral plexus, and it is made of the primary ventral rami of the first four lumbar nerves and a contribution of the subcostal nerve (T12), the last thoracic nerve. Multiple motor and sensory nerves are given off. The major motor branches consist of the femoral (L2-4) and obturator (L2-4) nerves. The major cutaneous, sensory branches consist of the iliohypogastric (L1), ilioinguinal (L1), genitofemoral (L1-2), lateral femoral cutaneous (L2-3), and anterior femoral cutaneous (L2-4) nerves. Most nerves are mixed motor and sensory. The intrinsic psoas nerves are the only purely motor nerves and the lateral femoral cutaneous nerve is the only purely sensory nerve.

2.1.1 Motor nerves

The femoral nerve is a mixed motor and sensory nerve that arises from the lateral border of the psoas muscle. It has two divisions, anterior and posterior. The anterior division gives off the anterior cutaneous nerve and muscular branches. It gives motor innervation to the pectineus and sartorius muscles. The posterior division gives off the saphenous nerve (sensory) and muscular branches. It gives motor innervation to the quadriceps femoris, which is composed of the rectus femoris, vastus lateralis, vastus medialis, and vastus intermedius.

The obturator nerve is a mixed motor and sensory nerve that arises from the medial border of the psoas muscle. It innervates the adductor muscles of the lower extremity. These include the external obturator, adductor longus, adductor brevis, adductor magnus, gracilis, and the pectineus (inconstant) muscles. It does not innervate the obturator internus. It also supplies the sensory innervation of the skin of the medial aspect of the proximal thigh.

2.1.2 Sensory nerves

The ilioinguinal nerve innervates the skin at the base of the penis and upper scrotum in males and the skin of the mons pubis and labia majora in females.

The iliohypogastric nerve consists of two branches that innervate the skin of the lower abdominal wall. The lateral cutaneous branch innervates the skin of the gluteal region. Of note, this nerve can also be injured when harvesting an anterior iliac crest bone graft. The anterior cutaneous branch innervates the hypogastric, or lower abdominal region.

The genitofemoral nerve consists of two branches, the genital and femoral branches. The genital branch innervates the cremaster muscle and scrotal skin in males and the skin of the mons pubis and labia majora in females. The femoral branch innervates the skin over the femoral triangle. This nerve is distinct from the other sensory nerves in that it does not follow a lateral trajectory to the site of innervation, but rather emerges on the anterior surface of the psoas and descends on the ventral surface.

The lateral femoral cutaneous nerve innervates the lateral aspect of the thigh. It consists of an anterior and a posterior branch. The anterior branch innervates the skin of the anterior and lateral surfaces of the thigh, as far as the knee. The posterior branch innervates the lateral and posterior surfaces of the thigh, from the level of the greater trochanter to the middle of the thigh.

The anterior femoral cutaneous nerve innervates the anterior and medial aspect of the thigh.

2.2 Safe zones

Early anatomic work related to the retroperitoneal transpsoas approach by Moro et al. helped to establish a safety zone to prevent nerve injuries when operating (Moro, et al., 2003). Specifically, they found that it was safe to traverse the psoas muscle at levels L4/5 and above, with the exception of the genitofemoral nerve, which is at risk at between L3 and L4.

Further studies described the course of the plexus, and found that the plexus lies within the substance of the psoas muscle between the junction of the transverse process and vertebral body, while exiting along the medial edge of the psoas distally (Benglis, et al., 2009). It is most dorsally positioned at the posterior endplate of L1/2 with a general trend of progressive ventral migration down to the level of L4/5. When a ratio of the distance from the posterior vertebral body wall to the total disc space length was calculated, it was found that there was a 0, 0.11, 0.18, and 0.28 ratio for L1/2, L2/3, L3/4, and L4/5, respectively. These findings suggest that an overly posterior placement of the dilator and/or retractor can lead to nerve injuries, especially at L4/5, where the ventral migration is nearly one third of the disc space from the posterior vertebral body wall.

A cadaveric study by Uribe et al. established four different zones and described safe working zones for MIS LIF (Uribe, et al., 2010) (Figure 1). The four zones represent different quartiles of the vertebral body, with zone I representing the most anterior and zone IV representing the most posterior quartile. The lumbar plexus, along with nerve roots, lie within the substance of the psoas muscle and dorsal to zone IV. The genitofemoral nerve was the only structure found to be ventral to zone III, starting at L2/3 and progressing caudally to L3/4 and L4/5.

It was determined that the safe anatomical zones to avoid nerve injury from L1/2 to L3/4 are the midpoint of zone III (posterior third of the disc space), and the safe zone for L4/5 is at the zone II/III junction (mid disc space). The genitofemoral nerve is at risk in zone II at

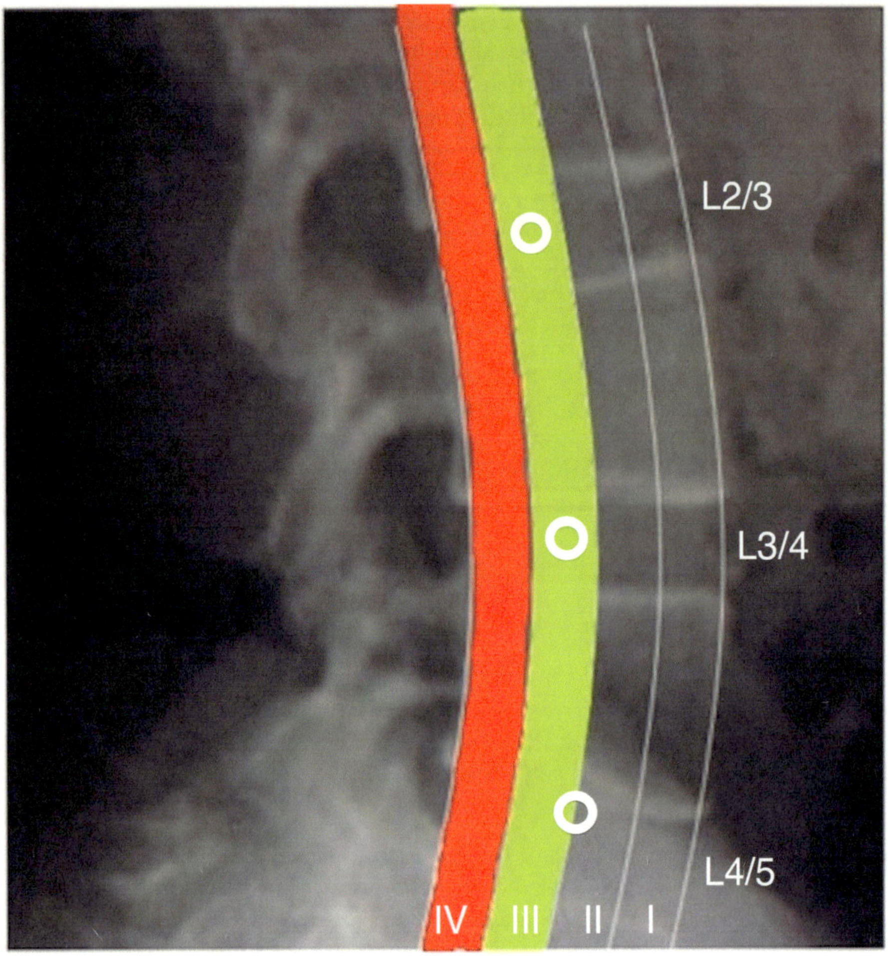

Fig. 1. Safe Anatomical Zones for MIS LIF. There are four quartiles, I-IV, from anterior to posterior. The open circles indicate a "safe zone" for placement of the retractor and for subsequent exposure. From L1/2 to L3/4, the posterior third is generally safe. At L4/5, placement at the midpoint between zone II and III is generally safe since this will decrease the risk of injuring the femoral nerve.

L2/3 and in zone I at L3/4 and L4/5. The ilioinguinal, iliohypogastric, and lateral femoral cutaneous nerves in the retroperitoneal space are also at risk since they travel obliquely, inferiorly, and anteriorly to the reach the iliac crest and the abdominal wall outside of the psoas in the retroperitoneal space.

There is a chance of lumbar plexus injury even in the early stages of the operation while obtaining access to the retroperitoneal space. Four nerves, the subcostal, iliohypogastric, ilioinguinal, and lateral femoral cutaneous nerves, are at risk of injury at this stage of the operation.

In addition to nerve injury, visceral and vascular structures should also be considered. The importance of meticulous preoperative planning was illustrated by Regev et al. in their morphometric study looking at the relationship of vascular structures as it relates to MIS LIF, where they found that the safe corridor for performing a discectomy and intervertebral cage placement progressively narrows from L1/2 to L4/5 (Regev, et al., 2009). In the presence of scoliosis, these corridors can potentially be further narrowed. One should also keep in mind that the kidneys are in the retroperitoneal space.

3. Surgical technique

The technique of the retroperitoneal transpsoas MIS LIF by our team has evolved with time and experience. Significant changes were made to our technique in 2010, and these changes have been the standard method we currently use for every patient. Specifically, the technique below refers to use of the XLIF® procedure. In general, the main principles apply to any lateral access system; however, a significant difference that will not apply to other systems is the use of a directional, triggered-EMG, which will be explained further in this discussion.

3.1 Preoperative planning and positioning

The preoperative planning is critical to ensure that the patient is a good surgical candidate. Preoperative magnetic resonance imaging (MRI) is evaluated to ensure that abdominal blood vessels will not hinder access to the desired disc space. A preoperative AP x-ray is evaluated to determine which side will provide the best access to the desired level, especially at L4/5, in relation to the iliac crest (Figure 2).

The patient is then placed in the lateral position with the optimal side facing up. If a scoliotic deformity is present, the patient is placed with the concave side facing up. The reasoning for this is that this usually provides better access to the L4/5 disc space if that it is an operative level. In addition, positioning the concave side up will allow for access to multiple levels through potentially fewer and smaller incisions.

At our institution, patients are placed on a Cmax® table (Steris, Mentor, OH), but any radiolucent operating table that allows for adjustment of flexion, extension, Trendelenburg/reverse Trendelenburg, as well as lateral tilting will suffice. The iliac crest is placed at the level of the table break where table flexion occurs. The legs are flexed maximally at the knee and hip to relax tension on the psoas muscle. A roll is placed beneath the axilla to prevent brachial plexus injury, and a roll is placed under the iliac crest to promote flexion at the iliac crest for improved access to the L4/5 level.

Intraoperative fluoroscopy is then used to position the patient in such a manner that a symmetric AP image with the pedicles equidistant from the spinous processes is achieved. It is essential that these images be as accurate and symmetric as possible to prevent inadvertently dissecting too far anteriorly or posteriorly. Caution should be exercised if a prior laminectomy exists over the desired level and spinous processes cannot be visualized.

Once properly positioned, the patient is taped and secured into place at the iliac crest and chest. The ipsilateral hip and leg are then taped to pull the iliac crest inferiorly and then secured to the table to prevent the patient from moving during surgery. The patient is then taped and secured into position (Figure 3).

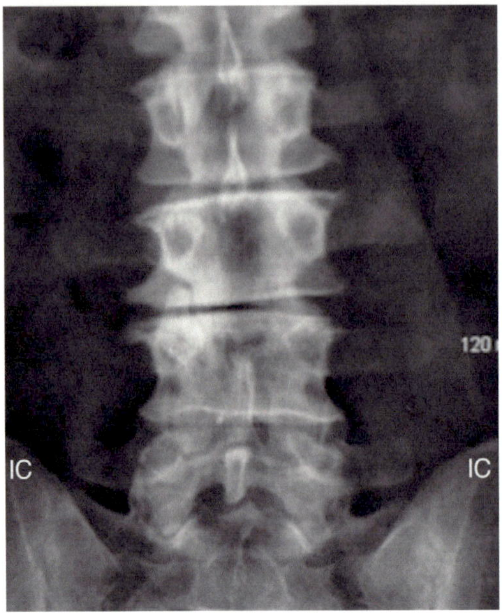

Fig. 2. AP radiograph of the Lumbar Spine. It is crucial to evaluate the clearance of the iliac crest (IC) preoperatively to determine positioning and operative feasibility.

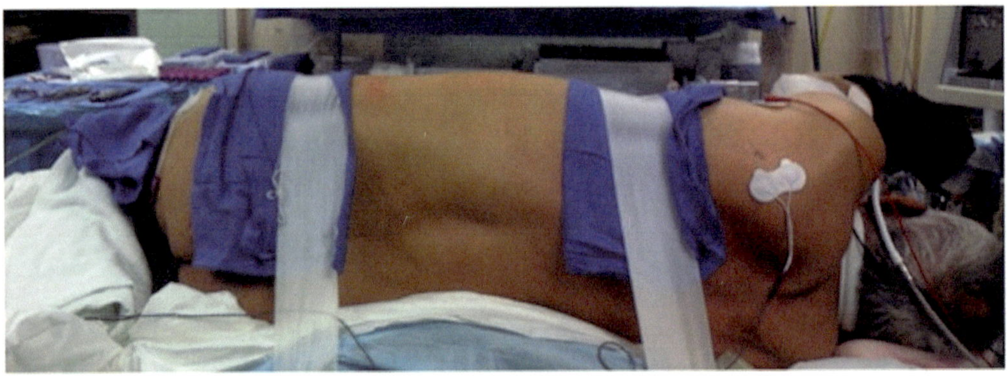

Fig. 3. Lateral Decubitus Positioning for MIS LIF. The patient is placed on an adjustable operative table and secured with silk tape. There is a bend in the table to allow for better access during surgery.

A repeat AP fluoroscopic image is again taken to ensure that good images are still obtainable and the bed is tilted slightly if correction of the image is needed. The relationship of the ipsilateral iliac crest and the lowest level to be approached are then evaluated. The angle of the disc space in relation to the iliac crest should ideally allow direct access to the disc space. At this point, the table is flexed at the level of the iliac crest just enough to give access to the disc space. If there is good access to the disc space without needing to flex the table, then it is advisable to perform the operation without flexing the table. Too much flexion of the table can put tension on the lumbar plexus and potentially cause nerve injury, so the table is flexed as minimally as possible while still achieving good access to the disc space.

Lateral fluoroscopy is then used, and the patient's position is modified with Trendelenburg or reverse Trendelenburg to obtain images clearly displaying endplates, posterior vertebral cortex, pedicle, as well as to evaluate the relationship of the disc space of interest to the ipsilateral iliac crest. A guide wire can be placed on the patient's skin to localize the plane of the disc space. Palpation of this area confirms that the iliac crest will not obstruct the pathway to the disc space.

An AP image for final positioning is then obtained to ensure there has not been any significant patient movement and that the images are still acceptable. Lateral fluoroscopy is then obtained to mark the disc space transversely and the posterior third of the disc space vertically. An exception is at L4/5, where the vertical mark is at the middle of the disc space based on the anatomic safe zones (Uribe, et al., 2010). If one level is to be approached, a single transverse incision approximately 5 cm is used. If more than one level is to be approached, a single vertical incision or multiple transverse incisions are used depending on the length of the incisions and cosmetic concerns.

3.2 Operative procedure

The area is then prepped and draped. An incision is made with a #10 scalpel blade to the subcutaneous fat. A second posterior incision is routinely not used as originally described (Ozgur, et al., 2006), as this route of access may cause injury to the ilioinguinal or iliohypogastric nerves (Uribe, et al., 2010). A self-retaining retractor is used to help dissect subcutaneous fat transversely along the original incision line with monopolar cautery until fascia is encountered. A transverse incision is then made in the fascia with monopolar cautery in line with the disc space. If multiple disc spaces are being approached, separate fascial incisions are made for each disc space to help stabilize the retractor.

Once the fascial incision over the area of interest is completed and muscle is encountered, two tonsil hemostats are used to dissect through muscle gently in the plane of the disc space through as small of an access as possible. Great care is taken to ensure the dissection is performed in line with the original skin marking for the posterior third of the disc space (or at the mid-vertebral body at L4/5) and that the dissection is not carried too anteriorly (to avoid bowel injury) or too posteriorly (to avoid nerve injury). The external oblique, internal oblique, and transversus abdominus muscles are identified and dissected until the transversalis fascia and retroperitoneal space are encountered.

Once in the retroperitoneal space, the quadratus lumborum can be palpated posterolaterally. The quadratus can then be followed medially until the transverse process of the vertebra of interest can be palpated. Then proceeding further medially, the psoas muscle can be palpated.

The first dilator can be inserted at this point, guided with the surgeon's finger anterior to the dilator to avoid peritoneal injury. The dilator is docked gently on the psoas without traversing the psoas. Lateral fluoroscopy is obtained to check position of the dilator to ensure it is in correct position (posterior third of the disc space, except for L4/5, in which case the middle of the disc space is the target) and the dilator position is adjusted as needed. The dilator is stimulated for triggered EMG (t-EMG) and the dilator is then rotated 360° to check for activity. Typically, anything ≥ 11 mA indicates a safe distance from any surrounding neural structure (Table 1). The dilator is then advanced through the psoas muscle until it is docked onto the spine. The dilator is again stimulated for t-EMG and rotated 360° to check for activity. Lateral fluoroscopy is again obtained to confirm position of the dilator in relation to the disc space as mentioned previously. If the stimulation of the initial dilator did not reveal any concerning t-EMG responses, a guide wire is placed through the dilator into the disc space to maintain position. Sequential dilators are then used to dilate the psoas muscle and stimulated in a similar fashion as described above. Once the final dilator is placed, it is stimulated for t-EMG and the responses are analyzed.

Numeric Reading (mA)	Color Displayed	Interpretation
≥ 11	Green	Acceptable
5-10	Yellow	Caution
< 5	Red	Alert

Table 1. Triggered EMG interpretation.

Sharp decreases in the threshold are not uncommon at this portion of the procedure. In fact, finding these sharp decreases are advantageous. The position of the femoral nerve can be estimated by the location of the sharp decreases in the t-EMG threshold. Ideally, the sharp decreases will be present when stimulating with the dilator posteriorly and increased thresholds present anteriorly; thus the femoral nerve can be estimated to be posterior to the dilators. This orientation will allow placement and opening of the retractor with minimal risk of nerve injury. If decreased thresholds are obtained anteriorly, the guide wire and dilators are removed and advanced more anteriorly so that the dilators are positioned anterior to the femoral nerve. The sequence for dilator and guide wire placement described above is again carried out.

Once the t-EMG stimulation with the final dilator verifies decreased threshold responses posteriorly and increased threshold responses anteriorly, the retractor is then placed over the dilators with the retractor blades oriented superiorly, inferiorly, and posteriorly. Downward pressure is applied to the retractor during the procedure until final placement of the shim blade to prevent psoas muscle fibers from creeping into the surgical field. The retractor is locked into place with the articulating arm while maintaining downward pressure. The dilators are removed while the guide wire is kept in place. A light source is attached to the inferior blade and used in conjunction with suction to visualize the disc space while maintaining downward pressure on the retractor. The surgeon should be able to visualize "red & white" indicating the disc space and small amounts of psoas muscle fibers that have crept into the surgical field. If only "red" is seen, then too much psoas muscle is in the field to visualize the disc space. If only "white" is seen, it is possible that the fascia of the psoas muscle has not been penetrated, which may cause the retractor to shift if it slides off the fascia during the procedure. The field is also inspected for evidence of nerves that could be injured with the procedure. Anything suspicious for being a nerve is stimulated with manual t-EMG to check for EMG activity. Sensory nerves will not stimulate with t-EMG, so a high index of suspicion must be maintained for an object that does not trigger EMG response.

Once it is confirmed that disc space is visualized and no nerves are present in the surgical field, lateral x-ray is obtained to check the position of the retractor in relation to the disc space. The shim blade is engaged into the posterior blade of the retractor but not deep into the disc space yet.

The retractor, while maintaining downward pressure, is adjusted into the correct position. The articulating arm is loosened and moving the retractor in relation to the guide wire helps to maintain proper orientation. Once proper position is attained on lateral fluoroscopy, AP fluoroscopy is used to show the superior-inferior relation of the retractor blades to the disc space. The shim blade is advanced into the disc space and malleted into position firmly with image guidance using AP fluoroscopy. The articulating arm is then attached and tightened to lock the retractor into position. Lateral fluoroscopy is then used to "look down" the posterior blade to ensure the proper pathway for the remainder of the procedure. The manual t-EMG stimulator is used to stimulate the entire surgical field and behind the posterior blade. Decreased thresholds elicited posterior to the posterior blade are expected and desired to ensure the working area is anterior to the femoral nerve, which is now protected by the posterior blade. The guide wire is then removed.

Once the retractor is in final position, the rest of the procedure must be performed as efficiently and quickly as possible to reduce the duration of retraction of the lumbar plexus. The retractor is now opened minimally to just allow discectomy and placement of the interbody graft.

The position of the anterior longitudinal ligament can be estimated by visualizing the slope of the anterior vertebral body. The procedure should remain as posterior as possible to this slope to prevent unwanted rupture of the anterior longitudinal ligament. A wide rectangular annulotomy is then made with an annulotomy knife. A pituitary rongeur is then used to remove disc material. A curved Cobb elevator is placed into the disc space with the handle vertically oriented and malleted under AP fluoroscopy guidance until the contralateral annulus is broken. This procedure is repeated with the curve of the Cobb elevator in the opposite orientation. The box cutter disc shaver is then placed in the disc space. Vertical orientation of the handle is confirmed and the box cutter is malleted flush with the posterior blade under AP fluoroscopy guidance to ensure the endplates are not violated. Once the box cutter is removed, AP fluoroscopy is used to confirm position of the shim blade in the disc space, which can be malleted into the disc space to guarantee the stability of the retractor. Again, a pituitary rongeur is used to remove disc material.

Depending on the preoperative x-ray, a straight or lordotic poly-ether-ether-ketone (PEEK) interbody cage can be filled with a variety of biologics. Our practice now is to pack approximately 5 cc of cadaveric cancellous bone mixed with mesenchymal stem cells (Osteocel Plus®, NuVasive, San Diego, CA) into the cage. A graft retainment device is used to retain the packed contents in the cage, and the cage is then placed in the disc space with a vertical orientation of the handle. It is malleted into position until the medial radiographic marker in line with the spinous process. The graft is then released and the retainment device removed. The surgical field is inspected for any graft that may have become dislodged during placement, and removed if idenified. The area is inspected for any bleeding and bipolar cautery can be used to obtain hemostasis. The articulating arm is loosened and the retractor is then closed. The retractor is removed slowly from the surgical field while inspecting for any bleeding.

Once the retractor is completely removed, final AP and lateral fluoroscopic images are obtained to ensure proper placement of the graft. The operating table is then leveled to assist with incision closure. Fascia is closed with interrupted 0 Vicryl sutures and the subcutaneous layer closed with 3-0 Vicryl sutures. The skin is approximated with 4-0 subcuticular Monocryl suture and dressed with Dermabond®.

4. Biomechanics

4.1 PEEK interbody cage

An essential component of MIS LIF is the placement of a large interbody cage. Traditionally, implant materials have been autograft or allograft bone, but issues with fracture, migration, and pseudoarthrosis led to the development of synthetic cages such as titanium, carbon fiber, and PEEK (Yang, et al., 2011). Among the synthetic cage materials, PEEK has been found to be favorable since it shares the same modulus of elasticity as bone (Brantigan & Steffee, 1993; Matge, 2002; Cho, et al., 2004). In addition, it is also non-absorbable, elicits a minimal cellular response, and allows for a clear, unobstructed view of new bone formation during follow-up exams (Boakye, et al., 2005; Vaidya, et al., 2008).

The placement of a large interbody cage, as accommodated by the lateral approach, is an advantage of MIS LIF. Large-diameter solid implants are less likely to subside compared to small-diameter cages, possibly related to a more efficient transfer of force to the endplate (Pearcy, et al., 1983; Closkey, et al., 1993; Lowe, et al., 2004).

4.2 Lateral plate

The MIS LIF can be supplemented with a lateral plate that spans across the disc space (Figure 4). The titanium plate has a rostral and caudal screw hole, and it can come in varying lengths (there is also a four-screw hole type, which we do not routinely use due to its larger profile). It is seated on two bicortical titanium screws that are placed across the width of the vertebral body parallel to the adjacent endplate.

Biomechanical comparisons between the lateral plate and stand-alone, unilateral pedicle screw, and bilateral pedicle screw constructs have demonstrated its increased rigidity compared to a stand-alone construct to promote arthrodesis (Bess, et al., 2008; Cappuccino, et al., 2010). The greatest biomechanical advantage of a lateral plate is its very favorable range of motion restriction in lateral bending, with only bilateral pedicle screws offering slightly more rigidity. In total, however, lateral plates still fall short of unilateral and bilateral pedicle screws, which are much more rigid overall.

Good candidates for a lateral plate supplementation should be free of any significant gross instability, since bilateral pedicle screws would be best in that situation. For similar reasons, lateral plates may not be optimal for deformity correction. In addition, bilateral pedicle screws are preferred in this situation because lateral plates only stabilize one segment at a time compared to multilevel stabilization offered by a unified, multilevel, pedicle screw and rod construct.

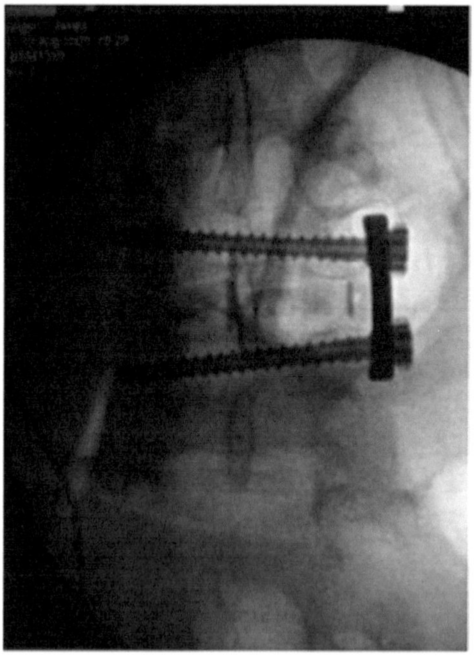

Fig. 4. Lateral Plate Fixation. This is an AP fluorographic view. Note the intervertebral cage placed spanning the entire vertebral body. The screws are placed near the subchondral bone.

5. Applications of the lateral approach

Surgical indications could include trauma, adult degenerative scoliosis, degenerative disc disease, spondylosis with instability, lumbar stenosis, spondylolisthesis, and adjacent segment failure. Early outcome studies have demonstrated that MIS LIF is associated with shorter OR times, minimal blood loss, few complications, minimal hospital length of stay, and quicker recovery (Dakwar, et al., 2010; Youssef, et al., 2010). Long-term outcomes are generally favorable, with maintained improvements in patient-reported pain and function scores as well as radiographic parameters, including high rates of fusion.

5.1 Degenerative spine disease and deformity

Minimally invasive techniques are increasingly used to treat degenerative spine disease and deformity. The factors that make MIS LIF appealing as mentioned above are an obvious draw to surgeons trying to minimize the morbidity associated with traditional open deformity correction (Carreon, et al., 2003; Okuda, et al., 2006). Using this technique, coronal Cobb angles can be improved (Anand, et al., 2010; Dakwar, et al., 2010; Tormenti, et al., 2010; Wang & Mummaneni, 2010) The effects on sagittal Cobb angles, such as with lumbar lordosis and the overall global sagittal balance, have not been as well established, however. This is an important topic since a positive global sagittal imbalance is most closely linked to a decreased quality of life, health status outcomes, and function (Schwab, et al., 2010). Sagittal imbalance can lead to higher energy requirements to stand and ambulate, leading to early fatigue, intolerance to standing, and walking with compensation through other joints.

The clinical outcomes data regarding deformity correction are encouraging thus far, with improved radiographic parameters as well as improved clinical results with a lower complication profile compared to traditional open approaches (Mundis, et al., 2010).

As the role of MIS LIF in spinal deformity correction is further clarified through further research, it is important to keep in mind that the ultimate end goal should still be to re-establish spinopelvic harmony, or the proportional relationships of one regional parameter to another as it relates to global spinopelvic alignment, as spinopelvic harmony has been directly linked to a satisfactory postsurgical outcome as assessed by health related quality of life instruments (Schwab, et al., 2010; Lafage, et al., 2011). Three basic radiographic targets to aim for in order to achieve spinopelvic harmony include: 1) sagittal vertical axis of < 50 mm or T1-SI < 0°, 2) pelvic tilt of < 20°, and 3) lumbar lordosis = pelvic incidence ± 9° (Schwab, et al., 2010). Attention to these three goals serve as the foundation for individual, patient-specific spinopelvic realignment in the sagittal plane, and even partial improvements of these parameters may translate to better clinical outcomes.

Adjacent segment failure is a common complication encountered in practice in patients with prior lumbar fusions. Operations to address this issue can often involve further posterior muscle dissection and revision of the existing instrumentation, all while negotiating through previous scar tissue, leading to risks of infection and CSF leaks. The MIS LIF is an option for treatment of adjacent segment failure. A virgin corridor is traversed, with placement of an intervertebral cage, which avoids some of the pitfalls of reoperations as mentioned above. In addition, if further internal fixation is desired, then a lateral plate could be placed without much additional difficulty. Literature regarding the specific use of the lateral retroperitoneal transpsoas approach is lacking for adjacent segment failure revision surgeries, but studies related to revision surgery using a this approach for revision and explantation of lumbar total disc replacements have shown its effectiveness and low rate of complications by avoiding a previous, scarred approach (Wagner, et al., 2006; Leary, et al., 2007; Patel, et al., 2008).

5.2 Trauma

Another area where there has been increased interest for the use of the lateral approach is trauma. Traumatic burst fractures commonly occur in the lumbar spine, with many occurring at the thoracolumbar junction. The decision of whether or not to treat with non-operative management with external orthoses or bedrest versus surgical decompression, instrumentation, and fusion is beyond the scope of this discussion. However, when surgical treatment is planned for situations where there is instability with neurologic deficit, a minimally invasive retroperitoneal transpsoas approach is an option.

In a report by Smith et al. with a follow-up of two years, patients treated with lateral corpectomies with supplemental instrumentation were found to have very favorable OR times, estimated blood loss, and hospital length of stay (Smith, et al., 2010). None of the patients required reoperations, and there was a significant improvement in the neurologic status based on the American Spinal Injury Association categorization, with none experiencing a neurologic decline.

6. Complications

As with any operation, there will always be a risk of complications that underscore the importance of meticulous attention to detail throughout the perioperative period (Knight, et al., 2009). Complications can arise from the result of inadequate preoperative planning. For instance, neurovascular structures may be in the way of the intended exposure, which may preclude a safe corridor for operating. Close attention to preoperative MRI's can help avoid this from happening. In addition, positioning mistakes leading to placement of the non-optimal side positioned up can make access to the L4/5 disc space, for example, much more difficult, leading to an increased risk of postoperative motor or sensory deficits.

6.1 Numbness, paresthesia, and weakness

The lateral retroperitoneal transpsoas approach is a technique that can be challenging since it is a non-traditional approach for many spine surgeons who are more accustomed to a posterior approach. Because of this, it does have a learning curve, and the skill at which it is performed is very dependent on experience with the regional anatomy and with the approach itself. Small changes in technique with this approach can result in dramatic changes in patient outcome due to the proximity of the lumbar plexus. Real-time EMG monitoring is critical to minimize the chance of motor nerve injury (Uribe, et al., 2010). However, sensory nerves cannot be monitored, thus leaving them susceptible to iatrogenic injury if there is not a thorough understanding of the regional anatomy.

Nerve injuries can lead to motor and sensory deficits, with the highest rates with L4/5 interbody approaches. The current literature is inconsistent with its reporting of postoperative "thigh" symptoms, which could range from numbness, paresthesias, dysesthesias, or weakness. Because of this, an overall rate of "thigh complications" ranging from 0.7% - 62.7% must be considered with a fair degree of caution (Knight, et al., 2009; Cummock, et al., 2011; Rodgers, et al., 2011).

When looking specifically at the type of complication, the rate of paresthesias following MIS LIF can range from 0.7% to 30% (Bergey, et al., 2004; Knight, et al., 2009; Cummock, et al., 2011; Rodgers, et al., 2011), and numbness has been reported in 8.3% - 42.4% (Dakwar, et al., 2010; Cummock, et al., 2011; Pimenta, et al., 2011). The specific nerve distribution may vary as well, but commonly affected nerves are the genitofemoral, lateral femoral cutaneous, and anterior femoral cutaneous nerves. It is important to distinguish between the different dermatomes of these sensory nerves on the postoperative examination, and not to simply report that a patient has thigh pain or numbness. Reports of motor weakness from femoral nerve injury have also varied, ranging from 3.4% - 23.7% (Knight, et al., 2009; Cummock, et al., 2011; Pimenta, et al., 2011).

It is important to realize that most motor and sensory deficits are transient and do recover, with 50% recovery at 90 days, and 90% recovery at 1 year (Cummock, et al., 2011). This may be a result of the muscles and nerves recovering from manipulation, inflammation, and irritation during the operation. As a result, it is advisable to fully disclose to patients preoperatively that there is a chance of motor or sensory deficit following the operation, but that the vast majority of cases are transient in nature.

6.2 Abdominal wall paresis

Abdominal wall paresis, also referred to as a "pseudohernia", has been identified as a potential complication of the MIS lateral approach (Dakwar, et al., 2011). The mechanism is attributed to iatrogenic nerve injury during the initial dissection of the abdominal wall. Consequences include denervation, paresis, and bulging of the anterior abdominal wall. Associated signs and symptoms include swelling, pain, hyperesthesia, or other sensory abnormalities. If suspected, it is important to rule out a true abdominal hernia in these instances. In many cases, spontaneous recovery can occur.

6.3 Hardware-related complications

There have been few reports of complications attributed to the hardware implanted such as the interbody cage or lateral plate. Recently, Dua et al. reported a 15% rate of hardware-related complications based off a series of 13 patients (Dua, et al., 2010). These cases consisted of two atraumatic coronal plane fractures at L4/5 in the first six weeks of the postoperative period.

A review of our own series has demonstrated a hardware-related complications rate of 5.9% in a series of 101 consecutive cases (Le, et al., 2011). The complications included three hardware failures and three vertebral body fractures. All cases were atraumatic. All cases presented with recurrent back pain except one, which was identified incidentally. All hardware failures involved a dislodged lateral plate and lock nut(s).

The mechanism is unclear, but may involve cage subsidence with a fixed angle screw, resulting in the screws cutting through the vertebral bodies in a coronal plane, a stress riser in the area of stress concentration, violation of the endplate during preparation or screw insertion, or malplacement of the hardware lock nuts (Disch, et al., 2008; Dua, et al., 2010; Le, et al., 2011).

6.4 Subsidence

As with any technique used for lumbar fusion, subsidence of the cage can occur at one or both endplates. The subsequent progressive deformity and compression of neural elements can lead to a loss of indirect decompression and reduced chance of successful fusion and possible reoperation (Closkey, et al., 1993; Kozak, et al., 1994).

In a study that included 140 patients and 238 levels fused in the lumbar spine with a mean follow-up of 9.6 months, we have recently found subsidence to be present in 14.3% of the cases, and in 8.8% of the total levels fused (Le, et al., 2011). Only 2.1% of the patients had symptomatic subsidence, however. Subsidence appears to correlate with construct length.

The most important finding, however, was that there was a 14.1% rate of subsidence with smaller 18 mm cages versus only 1.9% with larger 22 mm cages, leading to the conclusion that the largest interbody cage should be used whenever feasible.

6.5 Rhabdomyolysis

Rhabdomyolysis is a rare, but known, complication of spinal surgery. In severe cases, acute renal failure may result. The first cases of rhabdomyolysis and acute renal failure have recently been reported following MIS LIF (Dakwar, et al., 2011). This potential complication should be suspected in appropriate cases especially in morbidly obese patients and in procedures associated with prolonged operative times.

7. Conclusions and key points

The retroperitoneal transpsoas approach is a safe and effective alternative to traditional posterior, open lumbar techniques. It can be utilized for a variety of clinical applications including trauma, adult degenerative scoliosis, degenerative disc disease, spondylosis with instability, lumbar stenosis, spondylolisthesis, and adjacent segment failure. As with most minimally invasive techniques, there is a learning curve to be overcome in order to minimize the risk of iatrogenic nerve injuries. An integral aspect of this curve is to always be aware of the regional anatomy encountered. It is important to stay within the "safe zones" when performing an MIS LIF, staying in the posterior third of the disc space at L1/2, L2/3, and L3/4, or at the midpoint of the vertebral body at L4/5. Directional, t-EMG can help guide the surgeon and alert of any critical distances from surrounding motor nerves. Even with this, transient sensory deficits and, on occasion, weakness may occur, and it is important to discuss this potential with surgical candidates preoperatively.

8. References

Anand, N., Rosemann, R., Khalsa, B., & Baron, E. M. (2010). "Mid-term to long-term clinical and functional outcomes of minimally invasive correction and fusion for adults with scoliosis." Neurosurg Focus 28(3): E6.

Benglis, D. M., Elhammady, M. S., Levi, A. D., & Vanni, S. (2008). "Minimally invasive anterolateral approaches for the treatment of back pain and adult degenerative deformity." Neurosurgery 63(3 Suppl): 191-196.

Benglis, D. M., Vanni, S., & Levi, A. D. (2009). "An anatomical study of the lumbosacral plexus as related to the minimally invasive transpsoas approach to the lumbar spine." J Neurosurg Spine 10(2): 139-144.

Bergey, D. L., Villavicencio, A. T., Goldstein, T., & Regan, J. J. (2004). "Endoscopic lateral transpsoas approach to the lumbar spine." Spine (Phila Pa 1976) 29(15): 1681-1688.

Bess, R. S., Cornwall, G. B., Vance, R., Bachus, K. N., & Brodke, D. S. (2008). Biomechanics of lateral arthrodesis. eXtreme Lateral Interbody Fusion (XLIF). J. A. Goodrich and I. J. Volcan. St. Louis, Missouri, Quality Medical Publishing, Inc.: 31-40.

Boakye, M., Mummaneni, P. V., Garrett, M., Rodts, G., & Haid, R. (2005). "Anterior cervical discectomy and fusion involving a polyetheretherketone spacer and bone morphogenetic protein." J Neurosurg Spine 2(5): 521-525.

Brantigan, J. W., & Steffee, A. D. (1993). "A carbon fiber implant to aid interbody lumbar fusion. Two-year clinical results in the first 26 patients." Spine (Phila Pa 1976) 18(14): 2106-2107.

Cappuccino, A., Cornwall, G. B., Turner, A. W., Fogel, G. R., Duong, H. T., Kim, K. D., & Brodke, D. S. (2010). "Biomechanical analysis and review of lateral lumbar fusion constructs." Spine (Phila Pa 1976) 35(26 Suppl): S361-367.

Carreon, L. Y., Puno, R. M., Dimar, J. R., 2nd, Glassman, S. D., & Johnson, J. R. (2003). "Perioperative complications of posterior lumbar decompression and arthrodesis in older adults." J Bone Joint Surg Am 85-A(11): 2089-2092.

Cho, D. Y., Lee, W. Y., & Sheu, P. C. (2004). "Treatment of multilevel cervical fusion with cages." Surg Neurol 62(5): 378-385, discussion 385-376.

Closkey, R. F., Parsons, J. R., Lee, C. K., Blacksin, M. F., & Zimmerman, M. C. (1993). "Mechanics of interbody spinal fusion. Analysis of critical bone graft area." Spine (Phila Pa 1976) 18(8): 1011-1015.

Cloward, R. B. (1953). "The treatment of ruptured lumbar intervertebral discs by vertebral body fusion. I. Indications, operative technique, after care." J Neurosurg 10(2): 154-168.

Cummock, M. D., Vanni, S., Levi, A. D., Yu, Y., & Wang, M. Y. (2011). "An analysis of postoperative thigh symptoms after minimally invasive transpsoas lumbar interbody fusion." J Neurosurg Spine 15(1): 11-18.

Dakwar, E., Cardona, R. F., Smith, D. A., & Uribe, J. S. (2010). "Early outcomes and safety of the minimally invasive, lateral retroperitoneal transpsoas approach for adult degenerative scoliosis." Neurosurg Focus 28(3): E8.

Dakwar, E., Le, T. V., Baaj, A. A., Le, A. X., Smith, W. D., Akbarnia, B. A., & Uribe, J. S. (2011). "Abdominal wall paresis as a complication of minimally invasive lateral transpsoas interbody fusion." Neurosurg Focus 31(4): E18.

Dakwar, E., Rifkin, S. I., Volcan, I. J., Goodrich, J. A., & Uribe, J. S. (2011). "Rhabdomyolysis and acute renal failure following minimally invasive spine surgery: report of 5 cases." J Neurosurg Spine 14(6): 785-788.

Dakwar, E., Vale, F. L., & Uribe, J. S. (2011). "Trajectory of the main sensory and motor branches of the lumbar plexus outside the psoas muscle related to the lateral retroperitoneal transpsoas approach." J Neurosurg Spine 14(2): 290-295.

Disch, A. C., Knop, C., Schaser, K. D., Blauth, M., & Schmoelz, W. (2008). "Angular stable anterior plating following thoracolumbar corpectomy reveals superior segmental stability compared to conventional polyaxial plate fixation." Spine (Phila Pa 1976) 33(13): 1429-1437.

Dua, K., Kepler, C. K., Huang, R. C., & Marchenko, A. (2010). "Vertebral body fracture after anterolateral instrumentation and interbody fusion in two osteoporotic patients." Spine J 10(9): e11-15.

Eck, J. C., Hodges, S., & Humphreys, S. C. (2007). "Minimally invasive lumbar spinal fusion." J Am Acad Orthop Surg 15(6): 321-329.

Harms, J., & Rolinger, H. (1982). "[A one-stager procedure in operative treatment of spondylolistheses: dorsal traction-reposition and anterior fusion (author's transl)]." Z Orthop Ihre Grenzgeb 120(3): 343-347.

Harms, J. G., & Jeszenszky, D. (1998). "The unilateral, transforaminal approach for posterior lumbar interbody fusion." Oper Orthop Traumatol 6: 88-99.

Hodgson, A. R., & Stock, F. E. (1956). "Anterior spinal fusion a preliminary communication on the radical treatment of Pott's disease and Pott's paraplegia." Br J Surg 44(185): 266-275.

Knight, R. Q., Schwaegler, P., Hanscom, D., & Roh, J. (2009). "Direct lateral lumbar interbody fusion for degenerative conditions: early complication profile." J Spinal Disord Tech 22(1): 34-37.

Kozak, J. A., Heilman, A. E., & O'Brien, J. P. (1994). "Anterior lumbar fusion options. Technique and graft materials." Clin Orthop Relat Res(300): 45-51.

Lafage, V., Schwab, F., Vira, S., Patel, A., Ungar, B., & Farcy, J. P. (2011). "Spino-Pelvic Parameters After Surgery Can be Predicted: A Preliminary Formula and Validation of Standing Alignment." Spine (Phila Pa 1976) 36(13): 1037-1045.

Le, T. V., Baaj, A. A., Dakwar, E., Burkett, C. J., Murray, G., Smith, D. A., & Uribe, J. S. (2011). "Subsidence of PEEK Intervertebral Cages in Minimally Invasive Lateral Retroperitoneal Transpsoas Lumbar Interbody Fusion." Spine (Phila Pa 1976): In Press.

Le, T. V., Smith, D. A., Greenberg, M. S., Dakwar, E., Baaj, A. A., & Uribe, J. S. (2011). "Complications of lateral plating in the minimally invasive lateal transpsoas approach." J Neurosurg Spine: In Press.

Leary, S. P., Regan, J. J., Lanman, T. H., & Wagner, W. H. (2007). "Revision and explantation strategies involving the CHARITE lumbar artificial disc replacement." Spine (Phila Pa 1976) 32(9): 1001-1011.

Lowe, T. G., Hashim, S., Wilson, L. A., O'Brien, M. F., Smith, D. A., Diekmann, M. J., & Trommeter, J. (2004). "A biomechanical study of regional endplate strength and cage morphology as it relates to structural interbody support." Spine (Phila Pa 1976) 29(21): 2389-2394.

Matge, G. (2002). "Cervical cage fusion with 5 different implants: 250 cases." Acta Neurochir (Wien) 144(6): 539-549; discussion 550.

McAfee, P. C., Phillips, F. M., Andersson, G., Buvenenadran, A., Kim, C. W., Lauryssen, C., Isaacs, R. E., Youssef, J. A., Brodke, D. S., Cappuccino, A., Akbarnia, B. A., Mundis, G. M., Smith, W. D., Uribe, J. S., Garfin, S., Allen, R. T., Rodgers, W. B., Pimenta, L., & Taylor, W. (2010). "Minimally invasive spine surgery." Spine (Phila Pa 1976) 35(26 Suppl): S271-273.

Moro, T., Kikuchi, S., Konno, S., & Yaginuma, H. (2003). "An anatomic study of the lumbar plexus with respect to retroperitoneal endoscopic surgery." Spine (Phila Pa 1976) 28(5): 423-428; discussion 427-428.

Mundis, G. M., Akbarnia, B. A., & Phillips, F. M. (2010). "Adult deformity correction through minimally invasive lateral approach techniques." Spine (Phila Pa 1976) 35(26 Suppl): S312-321.

Okuda, S., Miyauchi, A., Oda, T., Haku, T., Yamamoto, T., & Iwasaki, M. (2006). "Surgical complications of posterior lumbar interbody fusion with total facetectomy in 251 patients." J Neurosurg Spine 4(4): 304-309.

Ozgur, B. M., Aryan, H. E., Pimenta, L., & Taylor, W. R. (2006). "Extreme Lateral Interbody Fusion (XLIF): a novel surgical technique for anterior lumbar interbody fusion." Spine J 6(4): 435-443.

Patel, A. A., Brodke, D. S., Pimenta, L., Bono, C. M., Hilibrand, A. S., Harrop, J. S., Riew, K. D., Youssef, J. A., & Vaccaro, A. R. (2008). "Revision strategies in lumbar total disc arthroplasty." Spine (Phila Pa 1976) 33(11): 1276-1283.

Pearcy, M. J., Evans, J. H., & O'Brien, J. P. (1983). "The load bearing capacity of vertebral cancellous bone in interbody fusion of the lumbar spine." Eng Med 12(4): 183-184.

Pimenta, L. (2001). Lateral endoscopic transpsoas retroperitoneal approach for lumbar spine surgery. VIII Brazilian Spine Society Meeting, Belo Horizo te, Minas Gerais, Brazil.

Pimenta, L., Oliveira, L., Schaffa, T., Coutinho, E., & Marchi, L. (2011). "Lumbar total disc replacement from an extreme lateral approach: clinical experience with a minimum of 2 years' follow-up." J Neurosurg Spine 14(1): 38-45.

Regev, G. J., Chen, L., Dhawan, M., Lee, Y. P., Garfin, S. R., & Kim, C. W. (2009). "Morphometric analysis of the ventral nerve roots and retroperitoneal vessels with respect to the minimally invasive lateral approach in normal and deformed spines." Spine (Phila Pa 1976) 34(12): 1330-1335.

Rodgers, W. B., Gerber, E. J., & Patterson, J. (2011). "Intraoperative and early postoperative complications in extreme lateral interbody fusion: an analysis of 600 cases." Spine (Phila Pa 1976) 36(1): 26-32.

Schwab, F., Patel, A., Ungar, B., Farcy, J. P., & Lafage, V. (2010). "Adult spinal deformity postoperative standing imbalance: how much can you tolerate? An overview of key parameters in assessing alignment and planning corrective surgery." Spine (Phila Pa 1976) 35(25): 2224-2231.

Smith, W. D., Dakwar, E., Le, T. V., Christian, G., Serrano, S., & Uribe, J. S. (2010). "Minimally invasive surgery for traumatic spinal pathologies: a mini-open, lateral approach in the thoracic and lumbar spine." Spine (Phila Pa 1976) 35(26 Suppl): S338-346.

Tormenti, M. J., Maserati, M. B., Bonfield, C. M., Okonkwo, D. O., & Kanter, A. S. (2010). "Complications and radiographic correction in adult scoliosis following combined transpsoas extreme lateral interbody fusion and posterior pedicle screw instrumentation." Neurosurg Focus 28(3): E7.

Uribe, J. S., Arredondo, N., Dakwar, E., & Vale, F. L. (2010). "Defining the safe working zones using the minimally invasive lateral retroperitoneal transpsoas approach: an anatomical study." J Neurosurg Spine 13(2): 260-266.

Uribe, J. S., Vale, F. L., & Dakwar, E. (2010). "Electromyographic monitoring and its anatomical implications in minimally invasive spine surgery." Spine (Phila Pa 1976) 35(26 Suppl): S368-374.

Vaidya, R., Sethi, A., Bartol, S., Jacobson, M., Coe, C., & Craig, J. G. (2008). "Complications in the use of rhBMP-2 in PEEK cages for interbody spinal fusions." J Spinal Disord Tech 21(8): 557-562.

Wagner, W. H., Regan, J. J., Leary, S. P., Lanman, T. H., Johnson, J. P., Rao, R. K., & Cossman, D. V. (2006). "Access strategies for revision or explantation of the Charite lumbar artificial disc replacement." J Vasc Surg 44(6): 1266-1272.

Wang, M. Y., Anderson, D. G., Poelstra, K. A., & Ludwig, S. C. (2008). "Minimally invasive posterior fixation." Neurosurgery 63(3 Suppl): 197-203.

Wang, M. Y., & Mummaneni, P. V. (2010). "Minimally invasive surgery for thoracolumbar spinal deformity: initial clinical experience with clinical and radiographic outcomes." Neurosurg Focus 28(3): E9.

Yang, J. J., Yu, C. H., Chang, B. S., Yeom, J. S., Lee, J. H., & Lee, C. K. (2011). "Subsidence and nonunion after anterior cervical interbody fusion using a stand-alone polyetheretherketone (PEEK) cage." Clin Orthop Surg 3(1): 16-23.

Youssef, J. A., McAfee, P. C., Patty, C. A., Raley, E., DeBauche, S., Shucosky, E., & Chotikul, L. (2010). "Minimally invasive surgery: lateral approach interbody fusion: results and review." Spine (Phila Pa 1976) 35(26 Suppl): S302-311.

Part 3

Surgical Approaches

7

Anterior Approaches to Thoracic and Thoraco-Lumbar Spine

Aydın Nadir
Department of Thoracic Surgery, Cumhuriyet University, School of Medicine Sivas-Türkiye

1. Introduction

Anterior surgical approaches have been used for lower cervical, thoracic, and upper lumbar vertebrae since the beginning of the second half of the 20th century. Hodgson et al. were the first surgeons to perform spinal fusion with anterior approach for the treatment of a paraplegic patient with Pott's disease in 1956. Cauchoix and Binet reported access to vertebral corpuses from C7 to T4 using a median sternotomy in 1957. Moreover, in 1969, Perot and Munro described trans-thoracic removal of a thoracic disc causing compression on the spinal cord. Similarly Dwyer et al. described the use of anterior approach for the surgical treatment of scoliosis (1969) and Harrington anteriorly stabilized vertebral fractures due to tumors with methyl methacrylate. First investigators to describe anterior approach with VATS were Mack et al. (1993) (1-4).

Surgical interventions for vertebral fractures include anterior, posterior and combined approaches, with the anterior approach providing a very good exposure. Posterior approach poses some technical inadequacy, with recurrence rates higher than the anterior approach. In fractures causing angle deformity, anterior approach has been proposed as the appropriate method. In fragmented fractures of the thoracolumbar spine, corpectomy with anterior approach and grafting is an effective treatment modality (2,5-8). Anterior approach not only provides a very good exposure to allow for decompression of the spinal canal, but also it may help to improve the neurological status in patients with neurological deficits. However, morbidity, which is mostly respiratory (atelectasis, respiratory failure, etc.), is more frequent with anterior approach (2).

Anterior approach was first reported by Dwyer and Zielke for scoliosis surgery, with a correction angle between 28,3°-66,6°. The average percentage of patients in whom correction can be achieved is 57.5%. Bilateral approach can be used or posterior approach can be combined with unilateral approach (1,3,9,10). In patients undergoing posterior surgery alone, the likelihood of requiring a second operation is high (11). In cases with scoliosis, the procedure should be performed at the side with widened intercostal spaces and convex deformity. When the thoracotomy is performed at the point of maximum deformity, better exposure is provided.

1.1 Indications

The primary indications for anterior approach in vertebral surgery include the conditions associated with the destruction of one or more vertebral corpuses and intervertebral discs, vertebral fractures, and deformities (**Table 1**). Whilst patients with deformities constitute the main patient population in childhood and adolescence, degenerative diseases, malignancies, and infections are the prevailing indications among adults. Recently, traumatic fractures with or without neurologic deficits also represent another very important indication for the anterior approach in spinal surgery. Pain relief, stabilization of the deformity, cosmetic improvement, drainage of spinal infections, and reduction/prevention of neurological deficits are primary objectives of such procedures (1,2,12,13).

Infection
Tuberculosis
Pyogenic infections
Parasitic infestation
Malignancy
Metastatic disease
Involvement by adjacent tumors
Primary tumor of vertebral body
Degeneratif disc disease (herniation)
Trauma
Fracture-dislocation
Compresion fracture
Spinal deformities
Scoliosis
Kyphosis
Lordosis

Table 1. Indications for anterior approach in spine surgery.

A multidisciplinary team effort involving thoracic surgeons, neurosurgeons, and orthopedic surgeons increases the likelihood of successful outcome with regard to operative results and improves the quality of life postoperatively. Inclusion of a thoracic surgeon in the team facilitates preoperative physiological assessments, determination of the best access route, and postoperative wound care (1,2).

1.2 Preoperative assessments

The preoperative assessment algorithm is the same as that is used for thoracic surgery. Pulmonary function tests and blood gas analyses are useful both for preoperative and postoperative care and evaluation of the cardiac status may help prevent postoperative complications (1,3,14,15).

Endotracheal general anesthesia with a single-lumen endotracheal tube is adequate for cervical (C7-T2) interventions, while endotracheal tubes with double-lumen should be preferred for thoracic and thoracolumbar procedures. Standard endotracheal tubes with a single-lumen may also be used. In our unit, tubes with a single-lumen are preferred. Retraction of the lung on the same surgical side without collapsing throughout the procedure will provide adequate exposure. This approach allows efficient use of time, and avoids some untoward occurrences such as malpositioning due to a double-lumen tube, inadequate aspiration, and intolerance to single-lung ventilation.

Appropriate positioning of the patient simplifies the surgery, shortens duration of surgery, and reduces the likelihood of morbidity. In cervical procedures the patient is brought to supine position, arms are adducted, and the head is slightly rotated toward the opposite side of the surgery. In case of open surgery between T2-12 or VATS, a standard lateral decubitus position is preferred. In our unit, we also prefer to use lateral decubitus position for anterior surgery in lower thoracic and upper lumber vertebrae during thoracoabdominal procedures. In this case, a backward angulation between 10°-15° toward the operation table provides better exposure.

Depending on the position of the lesion, four different anatomical levels may be defined as follows: C7-T2, T2-T6, T6-T12, T12-L3 or L4. For lesions between C7 and T2, the best approach consists of manubrium resection or partial sternotomy in addition to cervical resection, while right thoracotomy is appropriate for T2-T6 lesions. We prefer left thoracotomy starting from T3 level for traumatic vertebral fractures. Due to the close adjacency of the descending aorta, aortic mobilization may be required in anterior approaches at T3 and T4. In the upper thoracic levels between T2 and T6, thoracotomy should be performed at the same level with the lesion. Between T6-T12, procedures are performed via a left thoracotomy. At this level, thoracotomy at one or two level above the lesion may provide better exposure due to downward inclination of the ribs. For lesions between T12-L3, 4 a left thoracoabdominal approach should be undertaken. Removal of the 11th or 12th rib provides wider exposure. Particularly, removal of the 11th or 12th rib provides easy extrapleural access to L1-L4 (2,14,15).

Over a 7-year period (2004-2011), 67 patients (17 females, 50 males) were operated on using an anterior approach at our institution (2). The most indication for surgery was trauma fracture in 50 (75%) patients. Distribution of ethiologies of the patients according to access level was detailed in **Table 2**. Mean operation time was about 2 to 3,5 hrs, and estimated blood loss was approximately 1000 mL. Among the 67 patients operated via the anterior approach, we observed four postoperative complications. One patient had empyema postoperatively which was treated with tube thoracotostomy and irrigation. Another patient with vertebral tumor developed hemorrhagic drainage (1100 cc/24 h) during the early postoperative period which resolved with conservative treatment. In two patients, wound infection developed which were treated with debridement and suturation.

Remainder of this chapter, the procedures will be described detailed with operative pictures and drawings especially the "thoraco-lumbar" procedure.

1.3 Anterior approach to the cervicothoracic spine

Anterior approach at cervicothoracic vertebrae poses some difficulties associated with the local anatomy and requires a good deal of anatomical knowledge of the bony, ligamentous, muscular, and neurovascular structures of the upper thoracic access routes. Cervical resection, partial resection of the manubrium and clavicle and advances in the surgical instrumentation provide adequate exposure.

	Access level			
	T3-6	T7-10	T11-L3	**Total**
Etiology	n	n	n	**n**
Trauma	3	6	**41**	**50**
Tumor	1	**4**	1	**6**
Tuberculosis		**3**	1	**4**
Scoliosis	2			**2**
Hydatid cyst	3			**3**
Kyphosis	1			**1**
Kyphoscoliosis		1		**1**
Total	**10**	**14**	**43**	**67**

Table 2. Distribution of ethiologies of the patients according to access levels.

A neck incision parallel to the sternocleidomastoid and extending up to the suprasternal notch is made in addition to partial sternotomy reaching T4 level (**Figure 1a-b**).

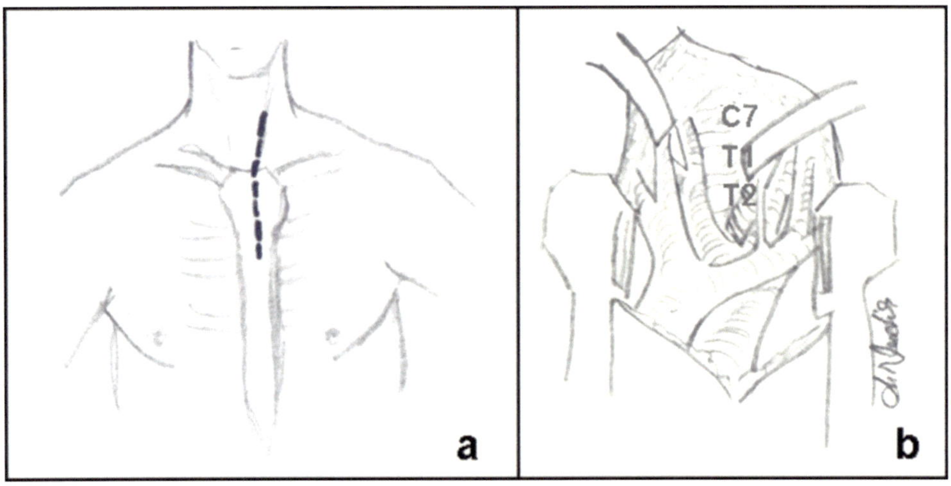

Fig. 1. Oblique neck and upper sternotomi incision is showing in figure 1a, and surgical exposure of C2 to T2 after the retraction of the vascular structures (Figure 1b). If clavicle is disarticulated form the manubrium, exposure can now be carried out to the T3.

A subplatysmal flap is prepared and strep muscles are pulled upwards to expose the sternoclavicular joint. Sternomastoid muscle is pulled laterally together with the jugular vein, and strap muscles are pulled toward medial side. Thus, the carotid sheath is positioned laterally, while the trachea and esophagus are positioned medially. Recurrent laryngeal nerve injury is avoided at the tracheoesophageal canal. Trachea and esophagus are pulled medially and the prevertebral fascia is exposed. Walsh et al recommend left sided neck incision due to decreased likelihood of injury to the contralateral laryngeal nerve, provided that there are no contraindications. Moreover, this approach provides better exposure from C4 to T3 (1,14,15).

Sternotomy may not be necessary to access T1 vertebra. In that case, partial excision of the manubrium and/or clavicle may provide adequate exposure. The sternocleidomastoid muscle is cut with cautery, strap muscles are divided and pulled upward, the sternal part of the pectoralis major is stripped toward lateral side, clavicle is stripped subperiosteally, and disarticulated from sternum. In this way, vascular structures are pulled more laterally. If required, inferior thyroid vein is ligated and manubrium is partially removed. A Hemovac drainage tube is placed into the operation area and the layers are closed in accordance with normal anatomic alignment.

1.4 Anterior Approach to the Thoracic Spine

The access route is determined by the spinal level and length of the procedure. In deformities such as scoliosis, a thoracotomy is performed at the side with the wider intercostal space where the deformity reaches its apex, which is defined as the most prominent site of deformity. When required, the rib at the level of the incision can be removed. Removal of the third rib provides a good exposure in T1-T4 lesions (1,2,6). Presence of the liver on the right side may result in technical problems; for this reason, we prefer left thoracotomy both for thoracic and lumbar procedures unless a contraindication exists. In situations such as the presence of a tumor or hydatid cyst, a left or right thoracotomy may be preferred depending on the location of the lesion (13,16-18).

After intubation in supine position, a lateral decubitus position with the left side on top is used. A skin incision from the appropriate intercostal space and extending up to paraspinal muscles is made and thoracotomy is commenced. Care should be experienced to provide congruity between the incision and the costal margin. The anterior edge of the latissimus dorsi is determined and cut by cauterization in the posterior direction. Serratus anterior is cut toward anterior direction starting from its posterior side along the ribs. The first rib is palpated under the scapula, ribs are counted, and intercostals muscles are cut at the preferred level and thoracic cavity is accessed. We do not perform rib resection in middle and lower thoracic procedures, since adequate exposure is achieved. If pleural adhesions are present, they are released by blunt or sharp dissection. In case of intubation with a single-lumen tube, a compression is placed upon the lung to provide mild compression. The parietal pleura is opened in cephalad and caudad directions. The perforating arteries from the aorta, if required, intercostal artery and vein are ligated and the vertebrae are accessed (**Figure 2**). Following the procedure, bleeding control is achieved and a 32F or 36F chest tube is placed in the pleural cavity before the layers are closed according to normal anatomical alignment. After a daily drainage volume of 50 to 100 ml and expansion of the lungs, the chest tube is usually withdrawn within 48-72 hours.

1.5 Anterior Approach to the Thoracolumbar Spine

Anatomy of the diaphragm is important for thoracolumbar approaches. The apex of the dome of diaphragm may reach T7 level. It is attached to the xiphoid bone anteriorly; to the ribs and costal cartilages laterally (ribs 6 to 12); and to the corpuses and transverse processes of L1, L2, and L3 vertebrae with the lumbosacral arch via the crura posteriorly. The right and left diaphragmatic crura reach the upper lumbar vertebrae by forming the aortic hiatus. Since the diaphragm is innervated centrally, the incisions on the diaphragm should be peripheral and circular.

The Adamkiewicz artery is the principal arterial supply to the spinal cord in the lumbar area and its injury leads to paraplegia. It arises from the intercostal artery from the left and right

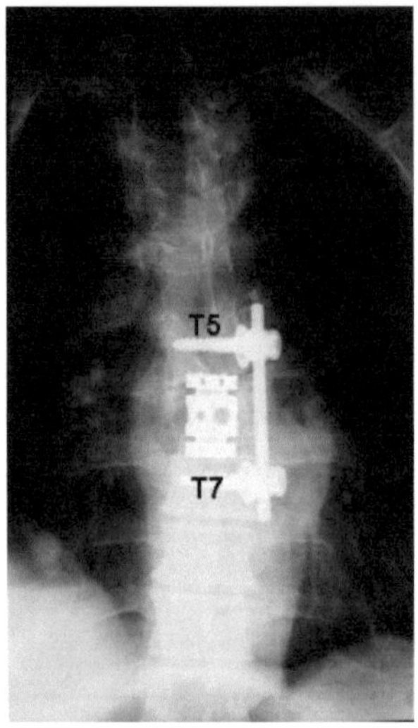

Fig. 2. The postero-anterior roentgenogram is showing fixating plates from T5 to T7 that is placed via left thoracotomy (Department of Neurosurgery, Cumhuriyet University, with permission).

side in 75% and 25% of the individuals, respectively (1,14,15). Maximum effort should be carried out to avoid injuring this artery in the critical vascular zone of the spinal cord, i.e. between T7-L4, and particularly between T8-T10. If required, a preoperative selective angiography may be helpful in deciding on the surgical approach and preventing paraplegia. Somato-sensory potentials monitoring is useful to minimize the risk of cordal ischemia, particularly when performing an anterior approach through the left side.

An incision along the 10th costal margin should be made for procedures between T10 and L1. In this regard, Hodgson recommends resection of the 9th rib, while Dwyer recommends the 10th. We prefer a transthoracic approach from the 9th intercostal space for T11-T12 lesions, while we access the thoracic cavity through the 10th intercostal space for T12-L1 lesions (2). For T12-L1, we access the retroperitoneal area with a transthoracic approach (**Figure 3a-b**). For the majority of cases this negates the need for costal resections. The diaphragm is stripped anteriorly-laterally over the vertebral corpus to reach L1 without disrupting the integrity of the diaphragm (**Figure 3,4**). If access to L2 is required in this approach, an additional circumferential resection 4 to 5 cm in length is made in the costal diaphragm. For L2 lesions, a resection at the 12th rib is performed to reach L1 L2 extrapleurally.

In lateral decubitus position, a posterior angulation of 10°-15° is provided for better exposure when the patient lies. In deformities such as scoliosis or kyphoscoliosis, the side of convexity is preferred for surgery. Otherwise, a left thoracotomy is performed based on simpler mobilization of the aorta and spleen as compared to inferior vena cava and liver. A skin incision along the appropriate costal margin is made and extended anteriorly toward the iliac crest. After the muscles are severed by cautery, ribs are accessed and removed up to the costal cartilage by deperiostization. Thoracic cavity is accessed. If access to L1 level suffices for the procedure, then diaphragm is stripped anteriorly-laterally without disrupting its integrity and the retroperitoneal area is accessed (**Figure 3-5**) without entering

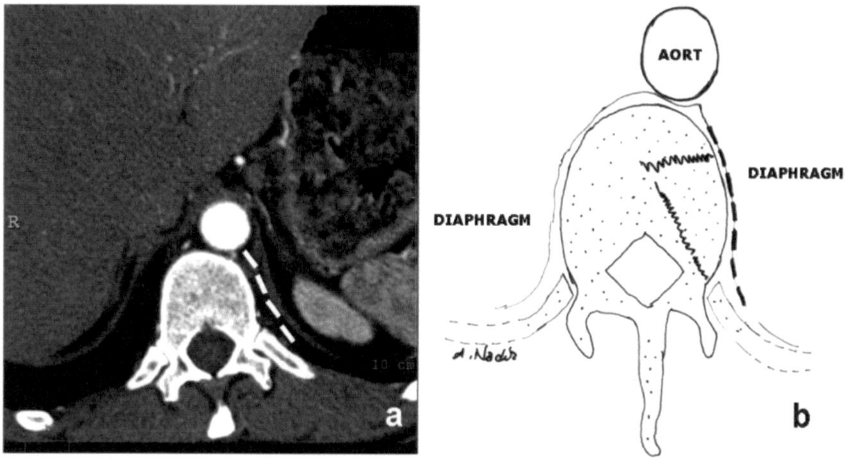

Fig. 3. The dotted lines showing the dissection plane either in radioloque (a), or schematic (b) illustration (The zig-zag lines in the b frame represents vertebral fractures).

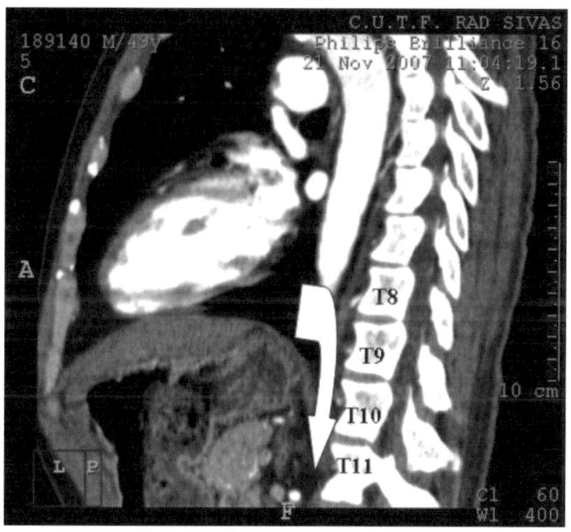

Fig. 4. White arrow indicating the pathway for reaching lumbal vertebrae during thoracotomy, in a sagittal section of a computed tomography. The diaphragm was separated from the antero-lateral vertebral corpus and the retroperitoneal space was reached without entering the abdomen, which allows access up to level L3.

the abdominal cavity. During the closure of diaphragm, infrequent sutures are usually adequate. Abdominal herniation is not expected, as only the retroperitoneal area has close association with the pleural cavity. In addition, the chest tube placed into the pleural cavity facilitates the postoperative drainage in the field of surgery.

For lesions at L2, a thoracoabdominal cut at the 11th or 12th costal region is performed (**Figure 6-9**). Removal of the 12th rib results in simple access to L3 (**Figure 10**), and if required, to L4. If necessary, lateral fibers of the abdominal muscles (external oblique, internal oblique, and abdominal transverse) can be opened carefully (14-16,19). Retroperitoneal area is reached without entering the pleural cavity. The porous tissues of the

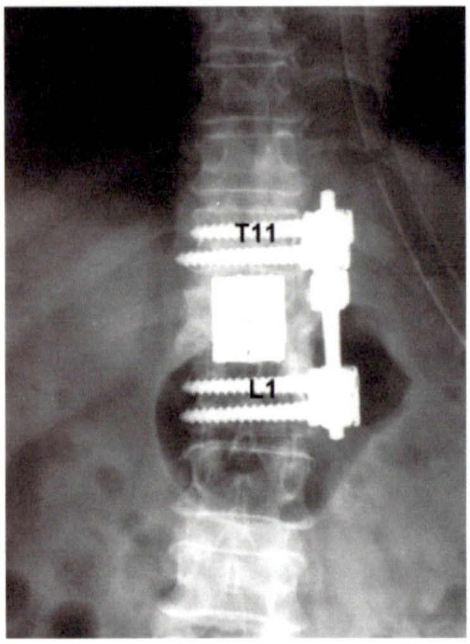

Fig. 5. The postero-anterior roentgenogram is showing the stabilization from T11 to L1. The diaphragm is divided from the vertebral corpus and reached the level L1 (Department of Neurosurgery, Cumhuriyet University, with permission).

retroperitoneum are retracted anteriorly and medially. The psoas muscle is stripped from its attachments to the L1 and L2 vertebrae using the vertebral column as a guide. Vertebrae are accessed. Sometimes thorax retractors may cause diaphragmatic injury, which can be closed by non-absorbable sutures for smaller defects. The lungs are fully expanded in coordination with the anesthesiologist. After absence of air in the pleural cavity is ascertained, the sutures placed on the diaphragm are ligated and the pleural cavity is closed without the need for a chest tube. Hemovac drains are placed in the field of surgery and under paraspinous muscles, and the layers are closed according to anatomy.

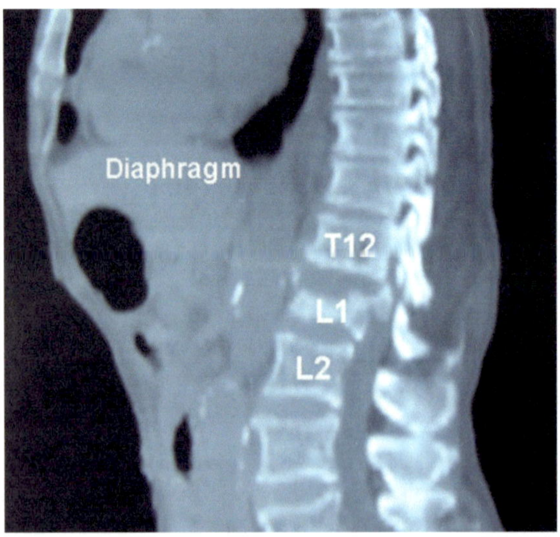

Fig. 6. The traumatic fracture in L1 vertebrae is revealed in the magnetic resonance imaging (Department of Neurosurgery, Cumhuriyet University, with permission).

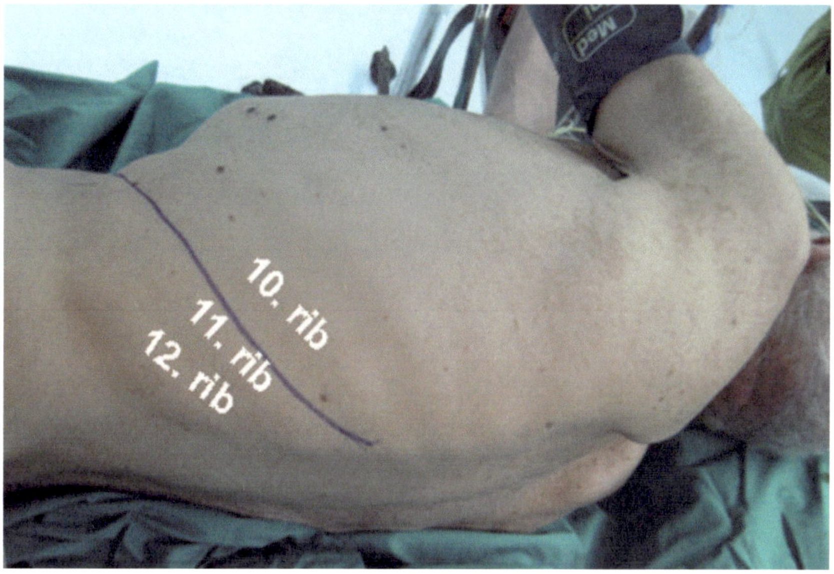

Fig. 7. The patient is placed in the lateral decubitus position with the left side up and is positioned in 10°-15° oblique chest position rotated to the posteriorly. The skin and subcutaneous tissue are opened from the lateral border of the paraspinous musculature to costal cartilage junction over the rib to be resected (Department of Neurosurgery, Cumhuriyet University, with permission).

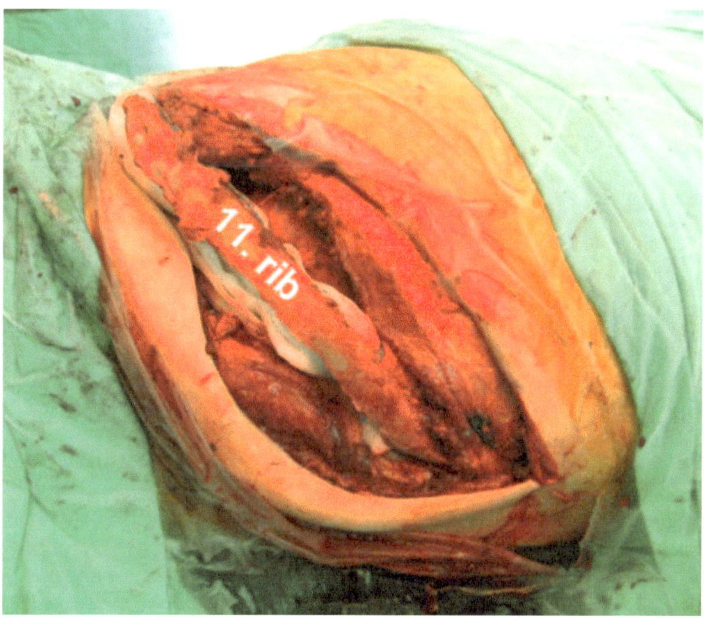

Fig. 8. The Periosteum is elevated first from the outer surface of the rib, then from the superior surface, followed by the inferior surface of the rib. The rib is cut as far anteriorly as between the costal cartilage junction and posteriorly at costotransverse joint (Department of Neurosurgery, Cumhuriyet University, with permission).

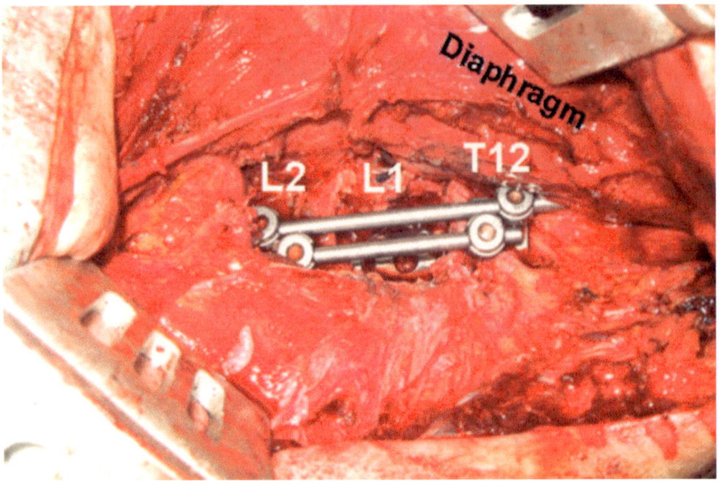

Fig. 9. Retroperitoneal area is accessed extrapleurally by the resection of 11th or 12th ribs depending on the location of the diaphragm. The intraoperative image of a patient following L1 corpectomy and stabilization by the aid of excellent exposure provided with the resection of 11th rib (Department of Neurosurgery, Cumhuriyet University, with permission).

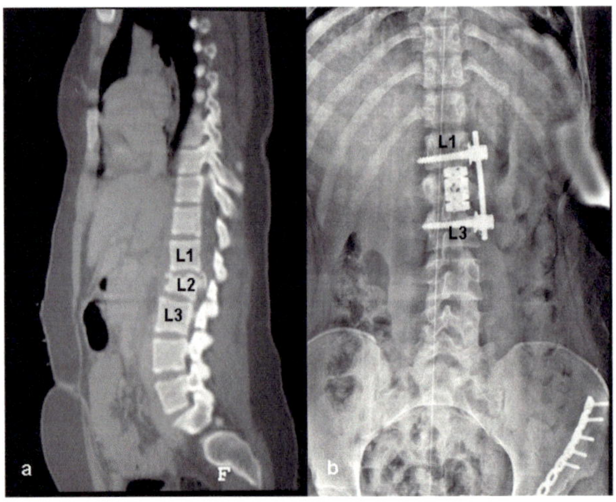

Fig. 10. Magnetic resonance imaging is showing traumatic vertebral fracture in L2 (a) and L2 corpectomy and stabilization was performed by the assistance with the resection of 12th rib (b) (Department of Neurosurgery, Cumhuriyet University, with permission).

Apart from the patients requiring vertebral resection due to metastasis of lung cancer, anterior approach with thoracotomy is required in spine surgery for conditions such as trauma, tumor, hydatid cyst etc. A good preoperative assessment of the vertebrae to be intervened is important for good exposure during surgery. Our experience showed us, thoracotomy levels should be placed according to the level of T6-7. If the lesion placed above that limit, then thoracotomy should be performed at the lesion point. If the lesion placed below that level, then thoracotomy should be performed one or two vertebrae higher than the lesion point.

2. References

[1] Mansour KA, DeLaRosa J. Anterior transthoracic approaches to the spine. In Shields TW, LoCicero J, Ponn RB, Rusch VW, ed. General Thoracic Surgery, vol 1, 6th ed. Philadelphia: Lippincott Williams and Wilkins; 2005:703-709.

[2] Nadir A, Sahin E, Ozum U, Karadag O, Tezeren G, Kaptanoglu M. Thoracotomy in spine surgery. Thorac Cardiovasc Surg 2008;56:482-84.

[3] Dwyer AF, Newton NC, Sherwood AA. An anterior approach to scoliosis. A preliminary report. Clin Orthop 1969;62:192.

[4] Levin R, Matusz D, Hasharoni A, Scharf C, Lonner B, Errico T. Mini-open thoracoscopically assisted thoracotomy versus video-assisted thoracoscopic surgery for anterior release in thoracic scoliosis and kyphosis: a comparison of operative and radiographic results. The Spine Journal 2005;5:632-8.

[5] Hitchon PW, Tomer J, Eichholz KM, Beeler SM. Comparison of anterolateral and posterior approaches in the management of thoracolumbar burst fractures. J Neurosurg Spine. 2006;5:117-25.

[6] Muschik MT, Kimmich H, Demmel T. Comparison of anterior and posterior double-rod instrumentation for thoracic idiopathic scoliosis:results of 141 patients. Eur Spine J 2006;1128-38.

[7] Schnee CL, Ansell LV. Selection criteria and outcome of operative approaches for thoracolumbar burst fractures with and without neurological deficit. J Neurosurg 1997;86:48-55.

[8] Denis F, Amstrong GW, Searls K, Matta L. Acute thoracolombar burst fractures in the absence of neurologic deficit: a comparison between operative and nonoperative treatment. Clin Orthop 1984;189:142-9.

[9] Liljengvist UR, Bullmann V, Schulte TL, Hackenverg L, Halm HF. Anterior dual rod instrumentation in idiopathic scoliosis. Eur Spine J 2006;15:1118-27.

[10] Jochen SH, Laurel B, Connie PK, George T. Video assisted thoracoscopic surgery in idiopathic scoliosis: evaluation of the learning curve. Spine 2007;32:703-7.

[11] Lapinsky AS, Richards BS. Preventing the crankshaft phenomenon by combining anterior fusion with posterior instrumentation. Does it work? Spine 1995;20:1392-8.

[12] Dai LY, Jiang SD, Wang XY, Jiang SY. A review of the management of thoracolumbar burst fractures. Surg Neurol 2007;67:221-31.

[13] Gurelik M, Goksel HM, Nadir A. Posterior mediastinal paravertebral hydatid cyst causing severe paraparesis. Br J Neurosurg. 2002; 16:605-6.

[14] Watkins R. Thoracic spine:anterior. In Herkowitz HN, Garfin SR, Eismont FJ, Bell GR, Balderston RA, ed. Rothman-Simeone Spine Surgery, vol 1, 5th ed, Philadelphia: Sunders Elsevier; 2006: 290-307.

[15] Thongtrangan I, Le HN, Park J, Kim DH. Thoracic and thoracolumar fractures. In Kim DH, Henn JS, Vaccaro AR, Dickman CA, ed Surgical anatomy&Techniques to the spine 9th ed, Philadelphia: Sunders Elsevier; 2006:352-363.

[16] Pettiford BL, Schuchert MJ, Jeyabalan G, Landreneau JR, Kilic A, Landreneau JP, Awais O, Kent MS, Ferson PF, Luketich JD, Peitzman AB, Landreneau RJ. Technical challenges and utility of anterior exposure for thoracic spine pathology. Ann Thorac Surg. 2008;86:1762-68.

[17] Lu DC, Lau D, Lee JG, Chou D. The transpedicular approach compared with the anterior approach:an analysis of 80 thoracolumbar corpectomies: clinical article. J Neurosurg-Spine 2010;12(6);583-591.

[18] Janik JS, Burrington JD, Janik JE, Wayne ER, Chang JH, Rothenberg SS. Anterior exposure of spinal deformities and tumors: a 20 year experienceJ Pediatr Surg 1997;32:852-9.

[19] Naunheim KS, Barnett MG, Crandall DG, Vaca KJ, Burkus JK. Anterior exposure of the thoracic spine. Ann Thorac Surg 1994;57:1436-9.

Part 4

Cervical Spine

8

Perforation Rates of Cervical Pedicle Screw Inserted from C3 to C6 - A Retrospective Analysis of 78 Patients over a Period 5 of 14 Years -

Jun Takahashi, Hiroki Hirabayashi, Hiroyuki Hashidate, Nobuhide Ogihara, Keijiro Mukaiyama, Syuugo Kuraishi, Masayuki Shimizu, Masashi Uehara and Hiroyuki Kato

Department of Orthopaedic Surgery, Shinshu University School of Medicine, Matsumoto-City, Nagano, Japan

1. Introduction

Cervical spine fixation using cervical pedicle screw (CPS) was first reported by Abumi [1] and Jeanneret [2] in 1994. Both reports described cases of cervical instability caused by cervical trauma. Cervical spine fixation by CPS was introduced as a procedure for the cervical instability of middle and/or lower cervical spine caused by trauma, and the importance of fixation by CPS for posterior cervical decompression and reconstruction was later reported [3,4]. Cervical pedicle screws can achieve rigid fixation compared to other cervical pedicle fixation methods [5, 6], and enable posterior cervical cord decompression. However, cervical pedicle screw insertion is technically demanding because of the narrow pedicle diameter and the risk of serious neurovascular complications including vertebral artery tear, spinal cord injury, and nerve root injury [7]. To achieve more accurate and safe pedicle screw insertion, navigation by two-dimensional imaging system or CT has been employed in recent years [9-12]. However, CPS insertion from C3 to C6 is technically demanding. The purpose of this study was to evaluate the perforation rates and direction of screw perforations in these insertions using CT-based navigation system.

2. Materials and methods

We evaluated 78 subjects (49 men and 29 women; mean age, 61.1 ± 14.2 years) who had undergone CPS insertion from C3 to C6 by using a CT-based navigation system from September 1997 to March 2011. A frameless stereotactic image-guidance system (StealthStation and Stealth Station TREON™; Medtronic, Sofamor Danek, Memphis, TN, USA) was used in screw placement and fixation of the cervical spine. The profile of cervical pedicle screw system was as follows; SUMMIT SI Occipito-cervico-thoracic (OCT) spinal fixation system (Depuy Spine, Inc., Raynham, MA), Olerud cervical system (Nord Opedic, Askim, Sweden), RRS Loop Spinal System (Robert Leid, Tokyo, Japan), Vertex Max system

(Medtronic, Sofamor Danek, Memphis, TN, USA) , Axon system (Synthes, Inc., West Chester, PA, USA), and Oasys (Optimal Aignment System) (Stryker Spine Allendale, NJ, USA).

Pedicle screw insertion technique assisted with navigation system

The basic data used for navigation were preoperative CT scan imaging data, consisting of consecutive axial slices 1 mm in thickness of the patients. The data were transferred to the system computer and were reconstructed into two-dimensional (2-D) and three-dimensional (3-D) images on a video monitor. Other mechanical components consisted of a computer workstation, a surgical reference frame, a probe rod to indicate the position in the surgical field, infrared light-emitting diodes (LEDs) that were attached to the probe rod, an electro-optical camera as a position sensor connected to the computer, and a drill guide. Infrared beams were tracked by the electro-optical camera system and the position of the respective LEDs was identified in real time in the surgical field.

Registration was performed in order to accurately match the computer-reconstructed 3-D surgical space with the real surgical space, by identifying four or more points on the vertebrae and the corresponding points of the vertebrae on the 3-D CT image on the monitor (matched-pair point registration). Though more precise matching of the two spaces is usually obtained by repeated registration procedures with 30 or more randomized points indicated by the probe on the surface of the vertebral body (surface registration), this group's procedure employs only 5 to 6 registration points for two consecutive lamina, to shorten the surgical time. More accurate positioning is possible by using the top of the spinous process and bilateral inferior facet caudal tip as points.

We established a surgical plan a day before surgery and confirmed insertion point of screws, applicability of 3.5 mm screws, point-for-point registration, screw position in relation to vertebral artery. This planning procedure took 20 to 40 min. Evaluation during the surgical plan for navigation provides further benefit by identifying pedicles with insertion risks and excluding such pedicles from operation (about 10% of all pedicles were excluded). Then, the entrance holes, direction, diameter, and depth of the screws were depicted with a cursor on the monitor, and the surgery was initiated. After exposure of the posterior bony elements of the spine, the reference frame was fixed to the spinous processes and the registration procedures described above were performed. After completion of the registration by matched-pair point and surface registration, the screws were inserted under the guidance of the navigation system. The position of the probe or drill guide was superimposed in real-time on CT images on the monitor, and the screws were introduced into the pedicles at the planned position indicated on the monitor. The required time between fixation of reference frame to spinous process and insertion of pedicle screw to each segment (1 or 2 vertebrae) was 10 to 15 min. After all screws were set, the reference frame for registration was removed and additional surgical procedures including decompression or bone graft were followed. If pedicle screw insertion was ineligible, sublaminar cable fixation by SecureStrand was performed.

Diseases included 22 cases (16 males, 6 females; mean age 52.2±18.8 years) of spinal trauma, 19 cases (8 males, 11 females; mean age 65.0±8.9 years) of rheumatoid arthritis (RA), 13 (7 males, 6 females; mean age 69.9±7.6 years) of cervical spondylotic myelopathy (CSM), 11 (7 males, 4 females; mean age 65.2±7.0 years) of destructive spondyloarthropathy (DSA), 6 (4 males, 2 females; mean age 62.3±9.1 years) of spine tumor, 5 cases (4 males; mean age 53.6±15.2 years) of cervical spondylotic myelopathy associated with athetoid cerebral palsy (CP), and 2 (2 males; mean age 45.5±10.6 years).

Using postoperative axial CT, the screw insertion status was classified as follows: grade 1 (no perforation), screw is accurately inserted in the pedicle; grade 2 (minor perforation), perforation of less than 50% of screw diameter; grade 3 (major perforation), perforation of 50% of screw diameter or more. The directions of perforations were evaluated as well.

The data were analyzed by a paired-sample Student *t* test using SPSS (SPSS Japan Inc., an IBM company, Tokyo, Japan), with $p<0.05$ defined as significant.

3. Results

Mean surgical time was 239±109 (range; 90 - 505) minutes. Mean blood loss volume was 352±327 (range; 20 - 1500) grams. For grade 3 (major perforation), the screw perforation rates by vertebral level were as follows: C3 (4/65, 6.2%), C4 (5/65, 7.7%), C5 (2/68, 3.1%), and C6 (1/76, 1.3%); therefore, higher perforation rates were observed for C4 and C3. For grade 3 and grade 2, the screw perforation rates by vertebral level were as follows: C3 (12/65, 18.5%), C4 (14/65, 21.5%), C5 (15/68, 22.1%), and C6 (8/76, 10.5%); therefore, higher perforation rates were observed for C5, C4, and C3, in this order (Fig. 1). For all the screws, the major perforation rate (only grade 3) was 4.4% (12/274) and perforation rate (grade 3 and grade 2) was 17.9% (49/274).

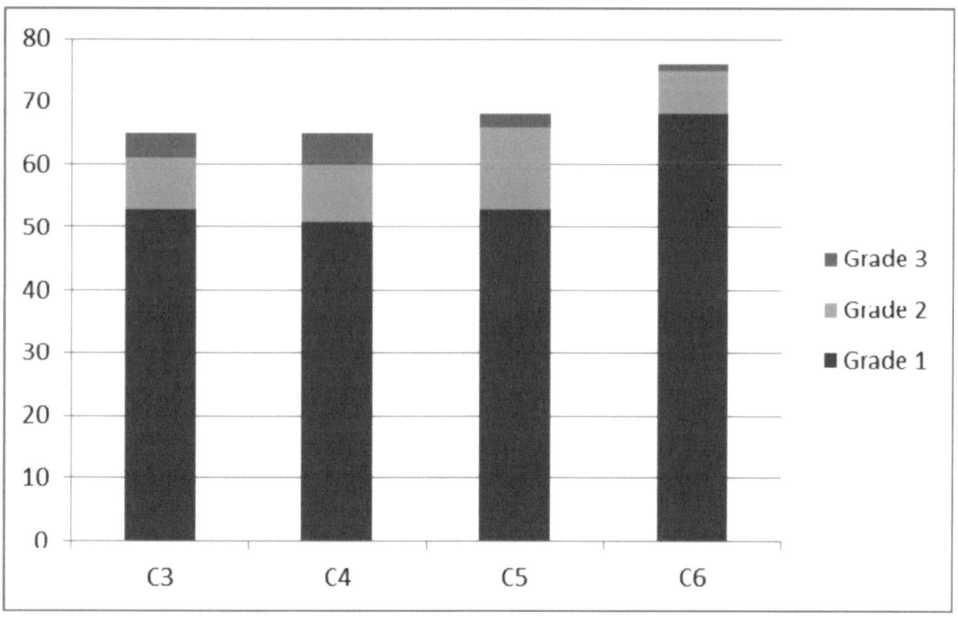

Fig. 1. Position of the cervical pedicle screw at different vertebral levels, observed by postoperative CT. Grade 1 (no perforation), screw is accurately inserted in the pedicle; Grade 2 (minor perforation), perforation of less than 50% of screw diameter; Grade 3 (major perforation), perforation of 50% of screw diameter or more.

The percentage of total lateral and medial perforations were 76% (37/49) and 24% (12/49), respectively. Grade 3 lateral and medial perforations were observed in 6 and 5 pedicles, respectively (Fig. 2). Grade 2 lateral and medial perforations were observed in 31 and 7 pedicles, respectively (Fig. 3). No vertebral artery tear, spinal cord injury, and nerve root injury were observed.

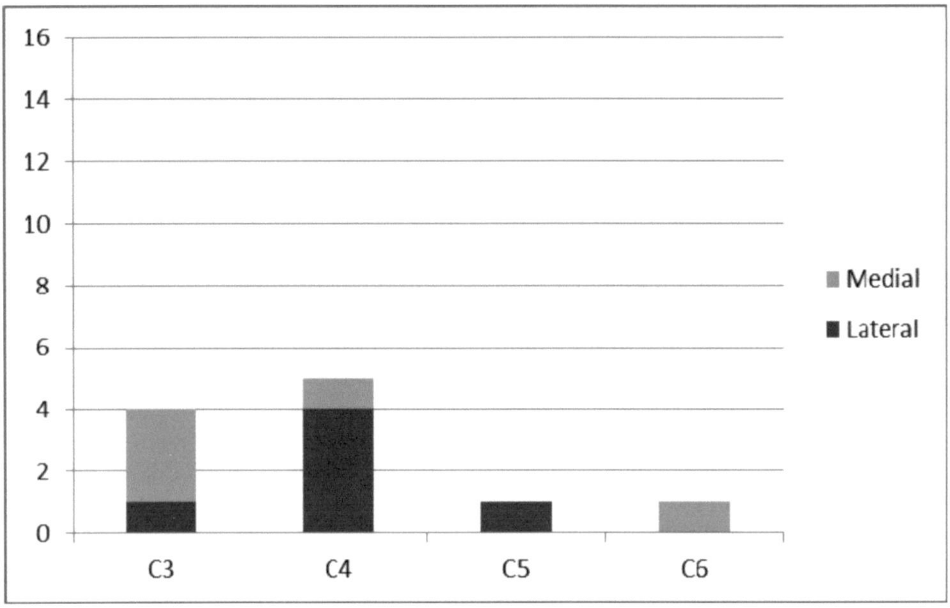

Fig. 2. Direction of grade 3 cervical pedicle screw perforation at different vertebral levels.

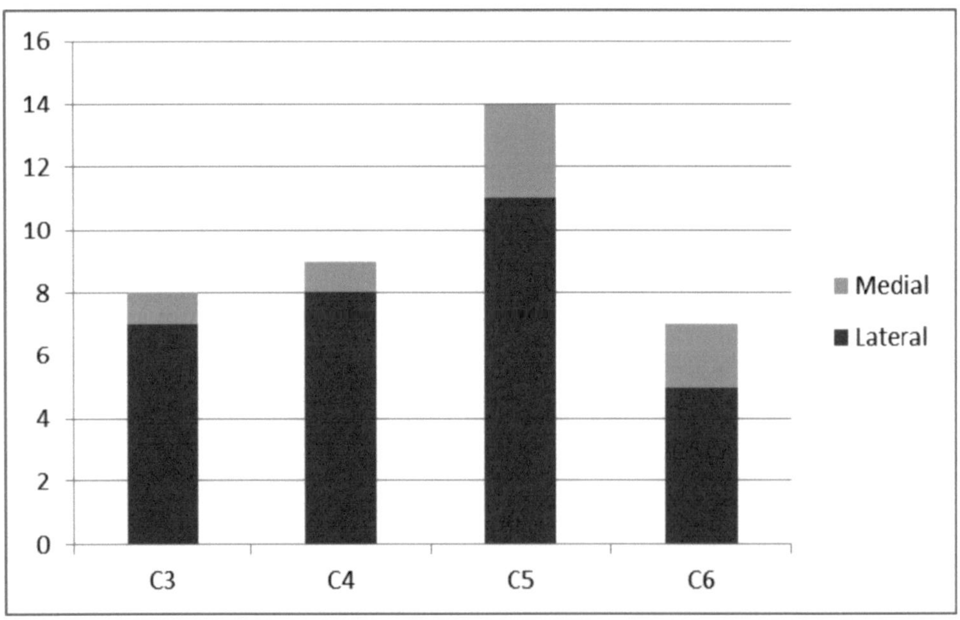

Fig. 3. Direction of grade 2 cervical pedicle screw perforation at different vertebral levels.

4. Case report

67 year-old male with rheumatoid cervical spine. The subject presented with spinal cord compression and instability at the C3-C4 and C4-C5 levels and showed myelopathy (Fig. 4) Laminoplasy and posterior fusion with CPS from C3 to C5 was performed (Fig. 5). Postoperative axial CT indicated the screw insertion status, which was as follows: bilateral C3, grade 2; right side of C4, grade 3; left side of C4, grade 2; and bilateral C5, grade 1 (Fig. 6).

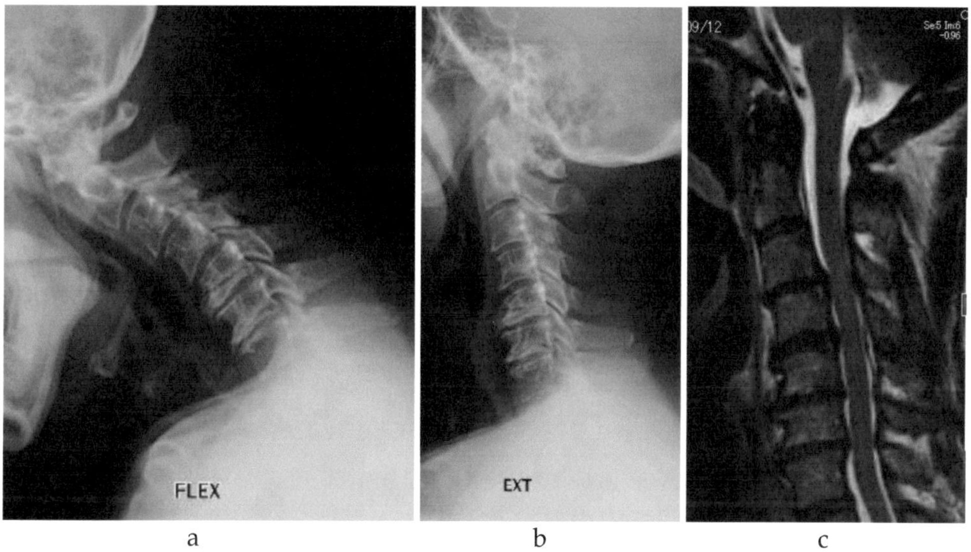

Fig. 4. a,b) Preoperative maximum flexion and extension lateral X-ray. Instability was observed at the C3-C4 and C4-C5 levels. c) MRI scan (T2-WI sagittal view). Spinal cord compression was observed at the C3-C4 and C4-C5 levels.

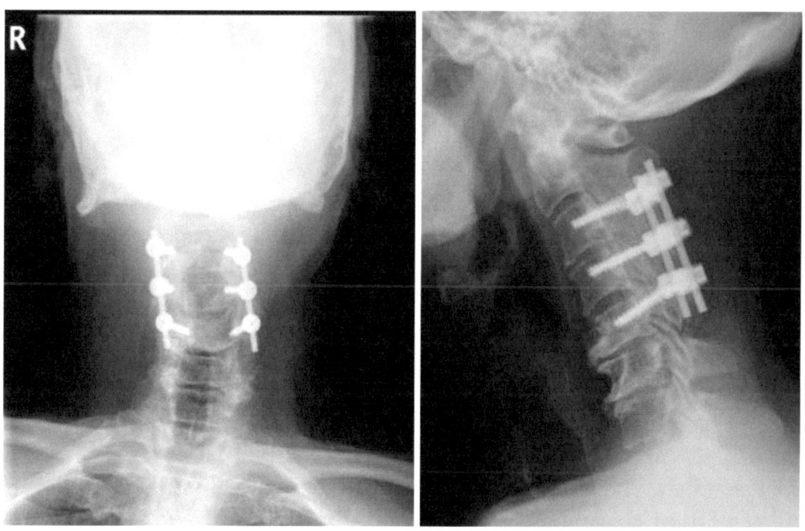

Fig. 5. Laminoplasy and posterior fusion with CPS from C3 to C5 was performed.

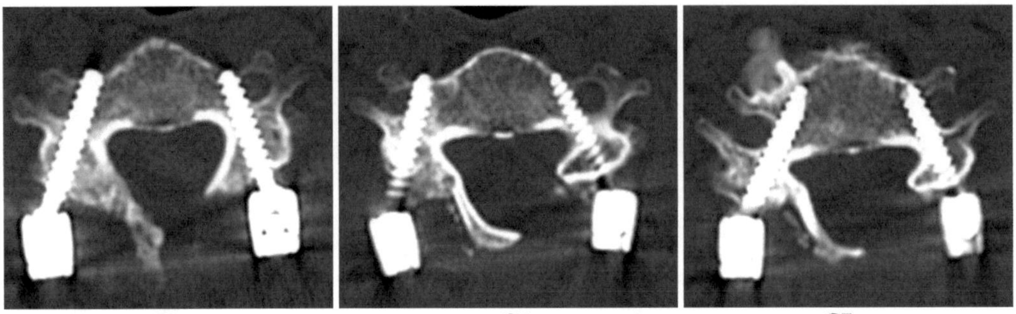

Fig. 6. Postoperative axial CT showed the following screw insertion status: bilateral C3, grade 2; right side of C4, grade 3; left side of C4, grade 2; and bilateral C5, grade 1.

5. Discussion

Cervical pedicle screws can achieve rigid fixation compared to other cervical pedicle fixation methods [13, 14], and enable posterior cervical cord decompression. However, cervical pedicle screw insertion is technically demanding because of the narrow pedicle diameter and the risk of serious neurovascular complications including vertebral artery tear, spinal cord injury, and nerve root injury [15]. Indication of cervical pedicle screw technique is as follows: destructive lesions including RA, DSA, and spine tumor; procedures that include both spinal cord decompression and posterior fusion. For rheumatoid cervical spine, this technique is especially useful because the strong initial fixation eliminates the necessity of postoperative external fixation such as halo vest or collar.

To achieve more accurate and safe pedicle screw insertion, navigation by two-dimensional imaging system or CT has been employed in recent years. In the meta-analysis reported by Tian et al., the accuracy of pedicle screw insertion by CT navigation (90.76%) was significantly improved compared to the two-dimensional imaging system (85.48%) [16]. Our institution employs a CT-based navigation system for the cervical pedicle screw insertion [9-12]. The result of this paper was that the percentage of major perforations were 4.4%, total perforation rates were 17.9% for all cervical pedicle screws. Richter et al. [17] reported comparative study of cervical pedicle screw fixation with conventional versus computer assisted surgery (CAS). In their result, pedicle perforation was 8.6% in conventional group and 3.0% in CAS group. Richter et al. indeed reported an excellent surgical outcome. The study of Richter et al. involved screw insertion for the upper thoracic vertebrae that have a larger vertebrae width as compared to the C3–C6 vertebrae that we studied, and vertebrae sizes could be larger in German individuals than in Japanese individuals. The reason for the larger perforation rate in our study could have resulted from the presence of a smaller pedicle in Japanese people and the narrow pedicle sizes of C3–C6 vertebrae.

Higher perforation rates for grade 3 (major perforation) were observed for C4 and C3. Furthermore, higher perforation rates for grade 2 and 3 (including minor perforation) were observed for C5, C4, and C3, in this order. For C6, the number of both major and minor perforations was small. Rheinhold et al. [18] measured the mean outer pedicle width for C3-C6 in human cadavers (mean age, 85 years), and the values for C3, C4, C5, and C6 were found to be 5.7 ± 0.4 mm, 5.6 ± 0.6 mm, 6.2 ± 0.6 mm, and 6.7 ± 0.6 mm, respectively. Yusof et al. [19] studied the transverse pedicle diameter of the C2-C7 of the cervical spine in a Malaysian population using computerized tomography (CT) measurements. The mean transverse diameters of the cervical pedicle of C3, C4, C5, and C6 in males were 5.2, 5.1, 5.2, and 5.5mm, respectively. In females, the mean transverse diameter of the cervical pedicle of C3, C4, C5, and C6 were 4.6, 4.7, 4.9, and 5.2mm, respectively. Our data on CPS perforation supported the results of the abovementioned studies in that pedicles with smaller diameters were found to have a larger number of perforations. The reason for the large number of minor perforations at C5 is unclear. C3 and C4 pedicles are generally narrow and hence, screw insertion is performed carefully. However, C5 is wider than C3 and C4; thus, the surgeon might be less attentive during the screw insertion for C5, which could contribute to this finding. Therefore, careful attention should be paid with respect to major perforations in the case of the C3 and C4 pedicles.

We found that a larger number of minor perforations occurred in the lateral direction than in the medial direction and that many major perforations were observed in the medial direction at the C3 level. During screw insertion in the cervical pedicle, the cortex is thicker in the medial direction and thinner in the lateral direction, and therefore, the CPS is likely to cause perforation in the lateral direction. In this study, perforation occurred in the lateral direction in 76% of the cases.

The possible causes of perforation of pedicle screw are as follows: Deviation of CT-based navigation system caused from unintentional movement of reference frame during operation etc.; lateral perforation caused by pressure from paravertebral muscle to probe, tap, or screw; narrow osteosclerotic pedicle that has no cancellous bone. To avoid perforation under such conditions, countermeasures as follows are required: If the practitioner judges the insertion point or screw direction shown by the navigation system is incorrect, intraoperative x-ray image or fluoroscopy shall be used. If screw direction could not be set sufficiently in the medial orientation, prepare a skin incision externally and insert probe, tap, and screw from the incision. In the case of narrow or osteosclerotic pedicle, skip the pedicle or change the fixation method to lateral mass screw, sublaminar cable, or other.

6. Conclusions

Major perforations were mostly observed in C4 and C3 pedicles. However, the number of C5 pedicle perforations was as large as C4 or C3 pedicle perforations when the total perforations, i.e., both major and minor perforations, were considered. The perforation rate of C6 pedicle was lesser than that for pedicles from C3 to C5. The major perforation rate for lateral and medial perforations was comparable. CPS insertion from C3 to C5 should be performed with extreme caution even under the CT-based navigation system.

7. References

[1] Abumi K, Itoh H, Taneichi H, Kaneda K. Transpedicular screw fixation for traumatic lesions of the middle and lower cervical spine: Description of the techniques and preliminary report. J Spinal Disord 1994;7:19-28.

[2] Janneret B, Gebhard JS, Magerl F. Transpedicular screw fixation of articular mass fractureseparation: Results of an anatomical study and operative technique. J Spinal Disord 1994;7:222-9.

[3] Abumi K, Kaneda K. Pedicle screw fixation for nontraumatic lesions of the spine. Spine 1997;22:1853-63.

[4] Abumi K, Kaneda K, Shono Y, Fujiyama M. One-stage posterior decompression and reconstruction of the cervical spine by using pedicle screw fixation systems. J Neurosurg 1999 ;90:19-26.

[5] Jones EI, Heller JG, Silcox DH, Hutton WC. Cervical pedicle screws versus lateral mass screws: Anatomic feasibility and biomechanical comparison. Spine 1997; 22:977-82.

[6] Kotani Y, Cunningham BW, Abumi K, McAfee PC. Biomechanical analysis of cervical stabilization systems: An assessment of transpedicular screw fixation in the cervical spine. Spine 1994;19:2529-39.

[7] Karaikovic EE, Kunakornsawat S, Daubs MD, Madsen TW, Gaines RW Jr. Surgical anatomy of the cervical pedicles: Landmarks for posterior cervical pedicle entrance localization. J Spinal Disord 2000; 13: 63-72.

[9] Takahashi J, Shono Y, Nakamura I, et al. Computer-assisted screw insertion for cervical disorders in rheumatoid arthritis. Eur Spine J 2007;16:485-494.

[10] Yuzawa Y, Kamimura M, Nakagawa H, et al. Surgical treatment with instrumen- tation for severely destructive spondyloarthropathy of cervical spine. J Spinal Disord Tech 2005; 18: 23-8.

[11] Ogihara N, Takahashi J, Hirabayashi H, Hashidate H, Kato H. Long-term results of computer-assisted posterior occipitocervical reconstruction.World Neurosurg. 2010; 73: 722-8.

[12] Uehara M, Takahashi J, Hirabayashi H, Hashidate H, Ogihara N, Mukaiyama K, Ikegami S, Kato H. Perforation rates of cervical pedicle screw insertion by disease and vertebral level. Open Orthop J. 2010; 4: 142-6.

[13] Jones EI, Heller JG, Silcox DH, Hutton WC. Cervical pedicle screws versus lateral mass screws: Anatomic feasibility and biomechanical comparison. Spine 1997; 22:977-82.

[14] Kotani Y, Cunningham BW, Abumi K, McAfee PC. Biomechanical analysis of cervical stabilization systems: An assessment of transpedicular screw fixation in the cervical spine. Spine 1994;19:2529-39.

[15] Karaikovic EE, Kunakornsawat S, Daubs MD, Madsen TW, Gaines RW Jr. Surgical anatomy of the cervical pedicles: Landmarks for posterior cervical pedicle entrance localization. J Spinal Disord 2000;13:63-72.

[16] Tian NF, Xu HZ. Image-guided pedicle screw insertion accuracy: a meta-analysis. Int Orthop. 2009; 33:895-903.

[17] Richter M, Cakir B, Schmidt R. Cervical pedicle screws: conventional versus computer-assisted placement of cannulated screws. Spine 2005;30:2280-7.

[18] Reinhold M, Magerl F, Rieger M, Blauth M. Cervical pedicle screw placement: feasibility and accuracy of two new insertion techniques based on morphometric data. Eur Spine J. 2007 ;16:47-56.

[19] Yusof MI, Ming LK, Abdullah MS, Yusof AH. Computerized tomographic measurement of the cervical pedicles diameter in a Malaysian population and the feasibility for transpedicular fixation. Spine 2006;31(8):E221-4.

9

General Description of Pediatric Acute Wryneck Condition

Alexander Gubin
St. Petersburg State Pediatric Medical Academy, Russia

1. Introduction

At least 80 causes of torticollis have been documented in the literature [1]. Acutely developed torticollis may mask severe pathology requiring treatment including surgical one. First of all, it is necessary to rule out trauma as well as the destructive process of tumoral or inflammatory nature. General differential-and-diagnostic algorithms required for examination of children with torticollis have been proposed (Fig. 1).

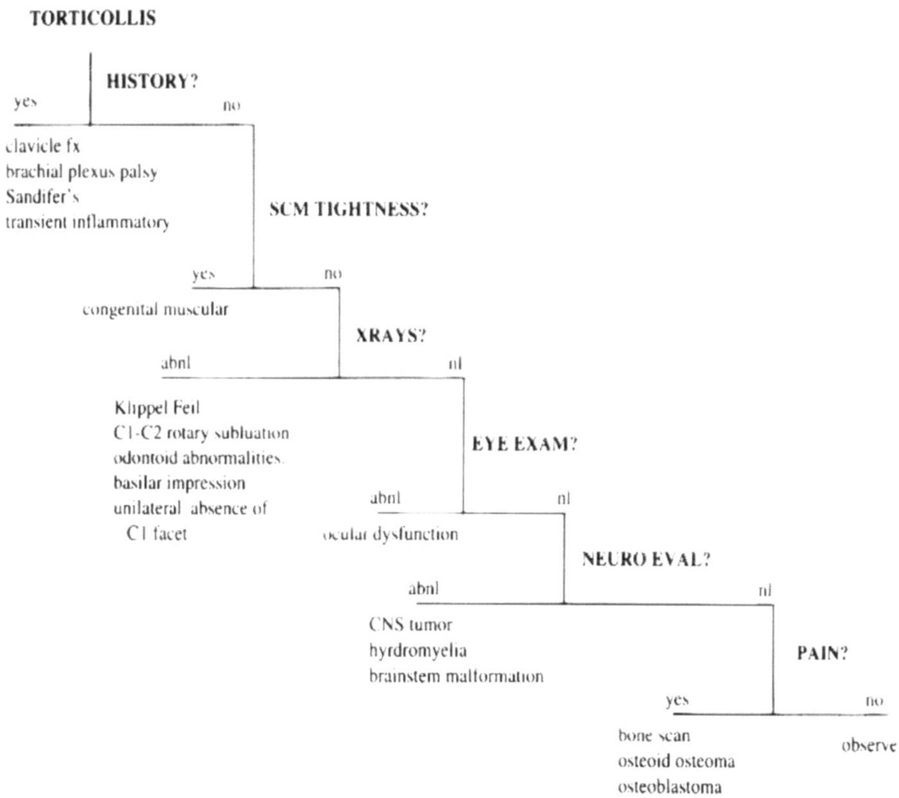

Fig. 1. Algorithm for examination of children with torticollis (cit. by [2]).

In case of acutely developed torticollis without traumatic effect the working diagnosis is made as acute torticollis or suspicion of rotatory subluxation, and in case of inflammation presence in nasopharynx it is made as the Grisel syndrome.

Such a child should be observed under out-patient conditions with prescription of immobilization and non-steroid anti-inflammatory medications. X-rays should not be made because torticollis prevents patient's proper positioning. In case of the pain syndrome and forced head position retention the patient should be hospitalized for examination and treatment. Thus, the acutely developed pathological head position and the pain syndrome in a child provided for ruling out traumatic and destructive causes is considered as a condition, the basis of which, according to most authors, is idiopathic atlantoaxial fixation or subluxation of CI.

Blankstein et al. (1997), who had analyzed the data of 33 patients over four years, found a clear seasonal trend – 58% cases accounted for the period from November to February, 33% of them – for the period from April to July [4]. Nemet et al. (2002) reported that 73% of cases in their group occurred in autumn and winter [5]. None of the authors mentioned could explain the phenomenon observed.

In our group (264 patients) the appearance of acute wryneck was the most characteristic for winter/spring period (70%). In the summer time mainly pre-school children were hospitalized with acute torticollis, while in the autumn children of the older school age prevail.

In majority of patients head side bending contra lateral to painful side has prevailed (Fig. 2). The «cock-robin position» with rotational motions block, classical for atlas-axial rotational subluxation description, is observed very rarely. Head side bending has varied from 10 to 45 degrees. The amount of rotational movements is restricted towards the painful side but had always prevailed over possibility for proper head positioning.

None of the authors tried to assess the pain syndrome intensity objectively. We found no attempts to connect the manifestation degree of the pathological head position with the characteristic features of x-ray picture. Despite the fact that some authors tried to characterize the range of motion in patients, it had no effect on the final diagnosis making or treatment character.

No relationship was found in the literature between the patient's age and the pain syndrome duration as well. In general, neck pain lasts from several hours to several days [5,6].

In our group minimal time needed to cut off pain syndrome is 24 hours; maximal one – is 10 days.

We've found the direct relationship between age of patients with acute torticollis and pain syndrome duration: the older a child, the longer is pain. So in children of babyhood the maximal duration of pain syndrome was 5 days and in older schoolchildren – 10 days.

With regard to neurological status, some authors consider complete neurological intactness [7] while others point to mild neurological symptoms as weakness in the limbs and headaches [4].

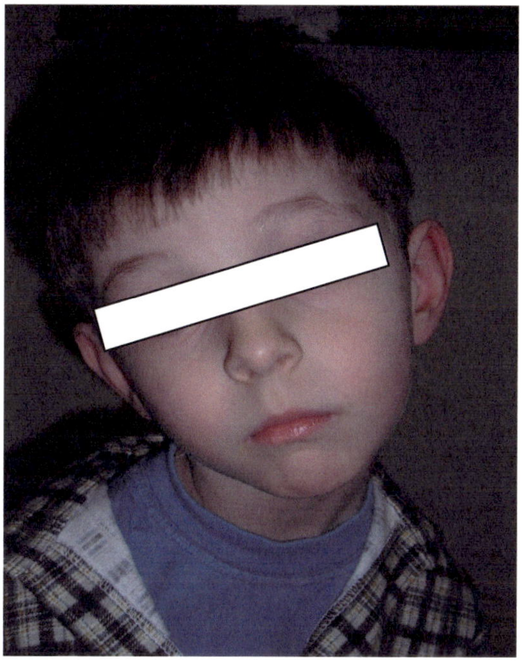

Fig. 2. Typical head position in a boy with wryneck.

2. Etiology and pathogenesis of acute torticollis in children

In N. Schwarz et al. opinion, the final decision on the direct pathogenetic cause of acute atlantoaxial rotatory subluxation (AARSL) in view of the current scope of scientific knowledge is difficult [8].

The inflammatory theory of CI subluxation was the principal until the middle of the XX century [9]. The Grisel syndrome was explained by the contracture of paravertebral muscles due to the pathological impulses from the focus of inflammation, or the inflammatory process dissemination to the lymph nodes behind the pharynx.

Most contemporary authors consider the Grisel syndrome cause as a direct inflammatory involvement of the soft-tissue structures of the atlantoaxial joint. The system of veins with frequent lymph-venous anastomoses between the periodontal venous plexus and the suboccipital epidural sinus may be a hematogenous intermediary to transfer the peripharyngeal inflammatory exudate to the zone of the atlantoaxial joint [10].

The theory of the entrapment of meniscoid bodies and torn ligaments in the cavity of the lateral atlantoaxial joints is more popular, and according to researchers it takes place for beyond-range rotatory motion of the neck with head tilt [11,12].

After performing a series of experiments on the anatomical preparations of atlantoaxial complexes with their subsequent freezing and making frontal and sagittal saw-cuts M.N. Nikitin (1965) put forward his theory [13,14]: «In case of uncoordinated movement of the head its lateral tilt occurs which leads to the expansion of the lateral atlantoaxial joint gap contralaterally, as a result of which the anterior and posterior parts of the joint capsule go deeply into the joint cavity as folds by 2/3 of the joint sagittal length at the expense of negative pressure (normally this hollow amounts to ½ of the joint sagittal length). The tension of the joint capsule lateral part, which occurs at that, causes irritation of nerve endings, thereby leading to reflex protective contraction of the muscles around the atlantoaxial complex, with entrapment of the capsule folds deepened and development of the joint blockade». This theory explains frequent beginning of acute AARSL from a sharp spasm of muscles during movements.

Another theory consists in atlas lateral mass getting on the side of its forward rotation to axis underlying part with joint gap overlapping (intervertebral blocking) [15-21]. This manifests itself as the radiological symptom of «winking». The coupling of the adjacent articular facets of the lateral atlantoaxial joints takes place in case of their getting (Fig. 3).

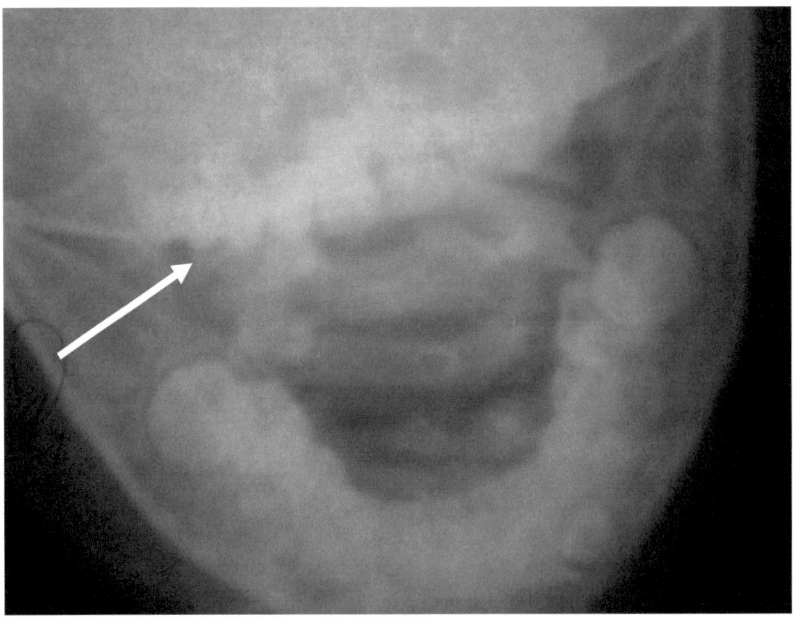

Fig. 3. «Winking» symptom in a child with AARSL. Marked CI-CII articulation locked (our case).

It should be noted that the analysis of the works demonstrating AARSL picture by dynamic 3-D CT confirms this point of view (Fig. 4).

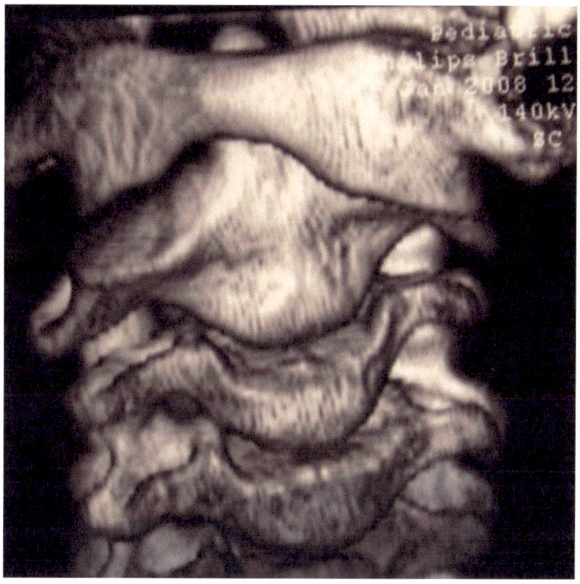

Fig. 4. 3-D CT of a child with AARSL. The getting of CI left articular surface to CII is clearly determined (our case).

The theory of acute muscular torticollis is considered in the literature as well. It is assumed that the pathological displacement of cervical vertebrae occurs due to muscle spasm [22].

The literature analysis allows to note that all the existing theories dealing with acute torticollis and AARSL development aside from intervertebral blocking are not confirmed by modern research methods (CT, MRI) and are the result of the authors' assumptions only. The lack of clarity in determining the causal relationships of all the theories proposed is not unimportant. No assumption clearly answers the question, what is the starting point for suffering beginning. Is CI subluxation the cause of the problem or its consequence ?

Maigne et al. (2003) have performed MRI of cervical spine in a 15-year adolescent in the early hours from the onset of typical acute torticollis developed after night sleep [23]. The authors did not rule out the disorder of CI-CII relation, but the signs of signal intensification were not found there. A hyperintensive wedge-shaped signal was determined by them in the zone of CII-CIII uncovertebral articulation on the side of pains (Fig. 5). It disappeared after three weeks by control MRI data. Torticollis quickly resolved by conservative treatment. The authors explained the finding by acutely occurred rupture of the intervertebral disc.

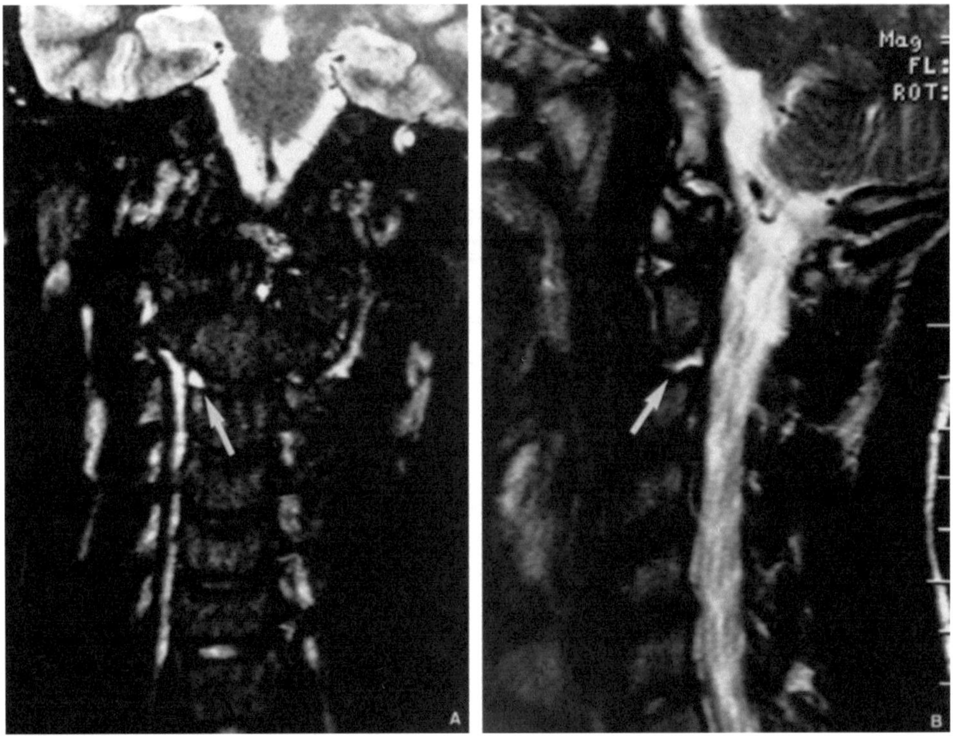

Fig 5. A hyperintensive wedge-shaped signal in the zone of CII CIII uncovertebral articulation (cit. [23]).

For identification of given pathological condition reasons we accepted a tactics of special MRI mode use in first hours after the patient's submission [24] .

We have made randomized sampling of patients with acute torticollis and atlas-axial block with a single selection criteria - first 12 hours after disease appearance. It has found to be reasonable for in 10 patients examined in succession, typical alteration were detected. They consisted in area of marked glowing of triangular or longitudinal shape in the area of external edge of C2-C3 or C3-C4 disk, and this glowing was always on the painful side (Fig. 6). The same findings that was presented by Maigne et al.

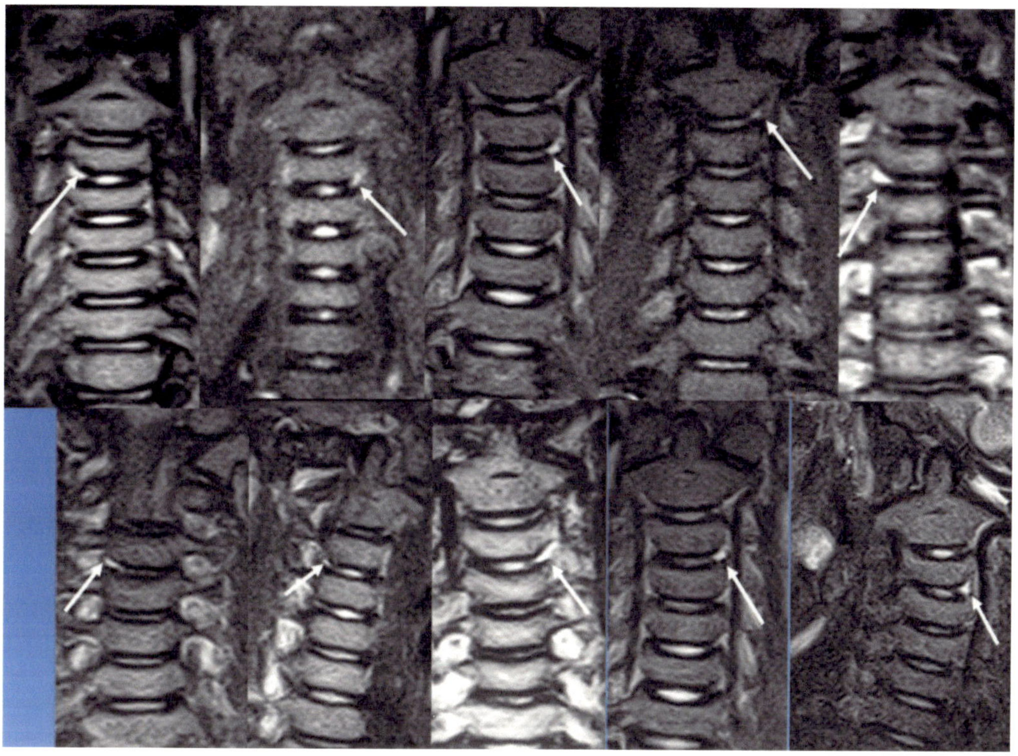

Fig. 6. MRI in the fat inhibition mode in 10 children with acute torticollis. The triangular area of hyperintensive signal is clearly seen in posterior-lateral parts of intervertebral space. The disk outline is separated from this area.

We propose the following mechanism of the syndrome development called "the uncovertebral wedge" [24,25]. Periosteal-facsial tissue in the area of uncovertebral joint is restricted by: hard borders of the disk fibrous ring from interiorly, posterior longitudinal ligament from posterior, hamus of caudal vertebra laterally and lamina of cranial vertebra from anterior. The reason of acute torticollis in children is in sharp or gradual compression of periosteal-facsial tissue in the uncovertebral fissure resulting from head movement or from long neck sidebending (sleep) with formation of a "wedge" from edematous tissue which irritates posterior longitudinal ligament. It leads to antalgic head position and, in some cases, to atlas-axial block. That's why traction reducing pressure in the uncovertebral fissure and contributing in venous drainage improvement and problem resolution is so efficient. Following arguments in favor of the given supposition seem to be equally important:

1. Uncovertebral joint is an exclusive anatomical neck specific, that's why similar conditions in children occur neither in lumbar nor in thoracic spine.
2. Pain appearance and its amplification in vertical posture, for here the pressure applied to intervertebral disk and correspondingly to uncovertebral "fissure" is increased.

3. Larger occurrence of acute torticollis in autumn/winter period may be explained by large amount of inflammatory alterations from the side of nasopharynx, that leads to venous drainage and adjacent tissue deterioration and edema complications.
4. Pathologically explainable becomes not only antalgic scoliosis (torticollis), but frequently observed kyphotic deformities in the cervical spine.

We suppose that age-related reduction and disappearance of acute torticollis and atlas-axial subluxations in adults is related to decrease of intervertebral disks resilience, to presence of powerful motion restrictors in the form of well-developed uncovertebral joints and to degenerative changes in Luschka joints.

3. Radiological findings in children with acute wryneck.

The vast majority of works deals with studying the atlantoaxial articulation X-rays. Some authors believe that the sign of asymmetric axis odontoid process location relative to atlas lateral masses is quite sufficient to make the diagnosis [26,27]. Others have doubts about the reliability of the most x-ray signs observed connecting them with the inability to achieve proper positioning in the process of x-ray study [28,29] or consider them as a variant of the norm [30]. While performing plane radiography Nicholson et al. (1999) reported that acute AARSL was not diagnosed in 67% of cases in their group of patients, and hyperdiagnosis had place in 29% of the cases [31]. That is to say, the radiological method has been recognized to be questionable in terms of assessing CI-CII relation for acute torticollis! Nevertheless, the most widely used classification of acute atlantoaxial rotatory subluxation has been proposed based on the clinical picture and radiological technique (Fig. 7). There are no Types III and IV in children.

The methods of dynamic radiography and cineradiography have not become popular because of the high level of radiation exposure [33].

The appearance of computer tomography in the 70-s of the XX century allowed researchers to define the details of atlas displacement more accurately [34-36]

At present dynamic and 3-D CT are mainly used [37]. Li et Pang (1995) have developed the criteria of 3-D dynamic CT using to define the diagnosis more exactly and develop the tactics for treating the atlantoaxial fixation [38]. They have refined the classification of Fielding J.W. et Hawkins R.J:

Type I - CI-CII is blocked with corrective rotation of the head;

Type II - CI-CII relation is improved with corrective rotation of the head:

Type IIA - CI-CII relation does not reach 0° with corrective rotation of the head;

Type IIB - CI-CII relation reaches 10° of rotation not more in the direction opposite blocking.

The more perfect tomography methods became and the more material collected, the more frequent were the data of the absence of visualization of the pathology in the atlantoaxial segment for the typical clinical picture of acute torticollis. Thus, Alanay et al. (2002) examined 15 girls and 21 boys at the age of 4-16 years with acute torticollis using dynamic CT, and they did not find the difference in CI-CII relations between them and normal children subjected to the similar study [39].

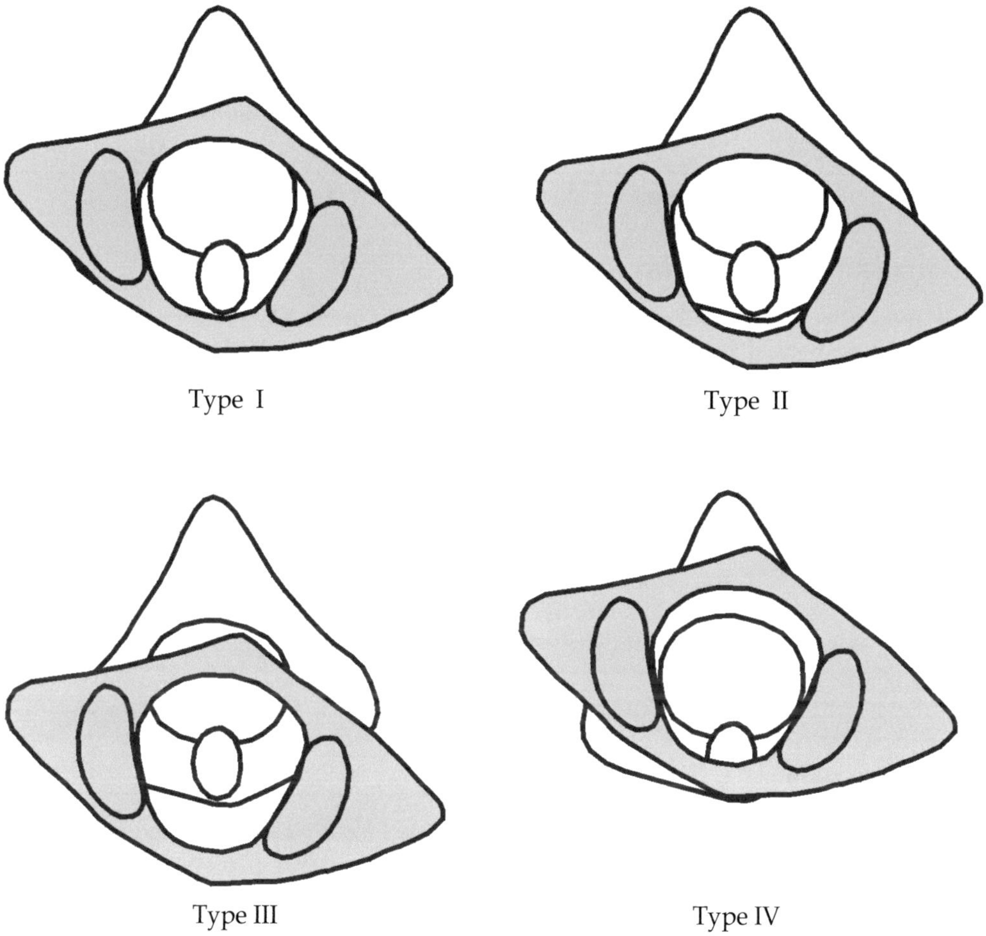

Type of acute AARSL	CI sagittal displacement	Size of Cruveilhier joint gap
Type I	Absent	3 mm
Type II	Anterior	3-5 mm
Type III	Anterior	› 5 mm
Type IV	Posterior	-

Fig. 7. Acute AARSL classification (cit. by [32]).

In the authors' opinion, there is no need to use dynamic CT in case of the fundamentally good-quality condition with spontaneous recovery which is represented by acute torticollis. They propose to use tomography in the cases of prolonged (more than one week) pain syndrome only. They have confirmed their first work by the second one with mathematical analysis and come to the same conclusions [40]. Other researches also had difficulties in the interpretation of CT picture for acute torticollis in children [41]. The main answer is absent in all the CT observations found in the literature: whether CI-CII relation disorder is a primary problem or a secondary positioning of the head. First of all, its use is justified for chronic AARSL [42].

Mainly MRI for torticollis is used to rule out a traumatic or destructive process [43].

4. Management of acute wryneck

Some authors within the end of the XIX century-first half of the XX century recommended to perform acute manual reduction for the purpose of subluxation elimination. The technique developed by Heister and Richet-Hueter was used for this purpose [44]. However, by the 60-s of the XX century this technique has lost its popularity, and most of the authors has recommended to perform loop traction.

The standard treatment regimen for patients with acute torticollis (suspicion of acute AARSL) has been reflected in most guides to Orthopedics (cit. by [3]):

1. Below one week: immobilization with soft collar, analgesics, bed rest; in case of recovery absence: hospitalization, traction;
2. Above one week, but below one month: hospitalization, loop traction, cervical collar for 4-6 weeks;
3. Above one month: hospitalization, skeletal traction, cervical collar for 4-6 weeks.

5. Conclusion

Children with sudden pain in the neck and constrained head position are frequent pediatric patients. It is reasonable to make a syndrome-related diagnosis on the stage of initial examination. The main task for a doctor is to separate those from the patients whose condition demands more profound examination, observation and treatment.

It is impossible to provide each patient with acute torticollis with full radiological examination and long observation in the hospital. That's why it is necessary to single out "danger levels" to provide this patients' group with adequate management [45]. We propose to single out 3 levels built by exclusion method (Fig. 8).

First level represents main flow of patients with multietiological and, in majority of cases, with "innocent" damages of cervical spine.

Second level represents patients with true atlas-axial subluxations demanding obligatory traction treatment to prevent pathology transition to chronic stage.

Third level includes patients with risk of mechanical and neurological instability demanding, as a rule, operative treatment. Besides usual injury it includes children with cervical developmental defects manifestation.

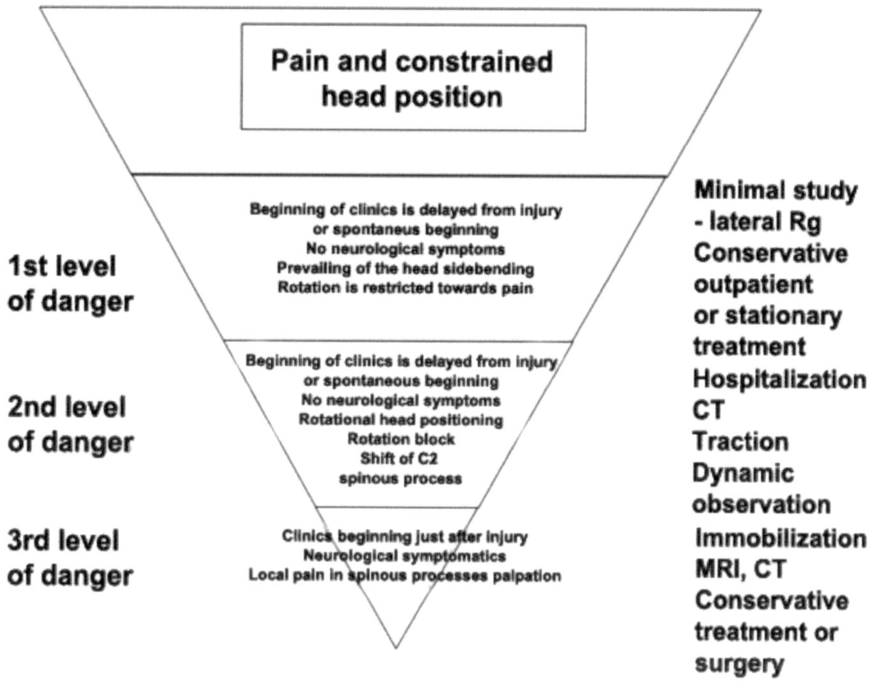

Fig. 8. Algorithm of surgeon's actions in case of admission of patients with acute pain syndrome and constrained head position. 3 incremental "danger levels". The pyramid narrowing to the 3rd level symbolically reflects amount of patients.

6. References

[1] Staheli, L.T. Practice of pediatric orthopedics / L.T. Staheli. - Philadelphia : Lippincot and Wilkins, 2006. - 460 p.

[2] Ballock, R. The Prevalence of Nonmuscular Causes of Torticollis in Children / R. Ballock, K. Song // J. Pediatr. Orthop. - 1996. - Vol. 16, N 4. - P. 500–504.

[3] Clark Ch.R. The cervical spine / Ch.R. Clark. - 4th ed. - Philadelphia : Lippincot and Wilkins, 2005. - 1250 p.

[4] Blankstein, A. Acquired torticollis in hospitalized children / A. Blankstein [et al.] // Harefuah. - 1997. - Vol. 133. - N 12. - P. 616–619.

[5] Nemet D. Acute acquired non-traumatic torticollis in hospitalized children / D. Nemet [et al.] // Harefuah. - 2002. - Vol. 141, N 6. - P. 519–521.

[6] Phillips, W.A. The management of rotatory atlanto-axial subluxation in children / W.A. Phillips, R. Hensinger // J. Bone Joint Surg. - 1989. - Vol. 71-A, N5. - P. 664–668.

[7] Subach, B.R. Current management of pediatric atlantoaxial rotatory subluxation / B.R. Subach, M.R. McLaughlin, A.L. Albright, I.F. Pollack // Spine. – 1998. – Vol. 23, N 20. – P. 2174–2179.

[8] Schwarz, N. The fate of missed atlanto-axial rotatory subluxation in children / N. Schwarz // Arch. Orthop. Trauma Surg. – 1998. – Vol. 117, N 4–5. – P. 288–289.

[9] Grisel, P. Enucleation de l'atlas et torticolis naso-pharyngien / P. Grisel // Presse Med. – 1930. – T. 38. – P. 50–53.

[10] Parke, W.W. The pharyngovertebral veins: an anatomical rationale for Grisel's syndrome / W.W. Parke, R.H. Rothman, M.D. Brown // J. Bone Jt. Surg. – 1984. – Vol. 66-A, N 4. – P. 568–574.

[11] Schwarz, N. Atlanto-axial rotation and distance in small children. A postmortem study / N. Schwarz, M. Lenz, A. Berzlanovich, W. Smetka // Unfallchir. – 2000. – Vol. 103, N 8. – P. 656–661.

[12] Vivas, I. Physiological rotatory C1-C2 subluxation in children / I. Vivas, J.L. Zubieta, C. Arriagada, C. Villas // Eur. Radiol. – 1999.- Vol 9 – P. 54.

[13] Никитин, М.Н. Об одной из причин ротационного подвывиха атланта / М.Н. Никитин // Ортопедия, травматология. – 1965. – № 4. – С. 47–52.

[14] Никитин, М.Н. Ротационные подвывихи атланта: дис. ... канд. мед. наук / Никитин М.Н. – Фрунзе, 1966. – 354 с.

[15] El-Khoury, G.Y. Acute traumatic rotatory atlanto-axial dislocation in children: a report of three cases / G.Y. El-Khoury, C.R. Clarc, A.W. Gravett // J. Bone Joint Surg. – 1984. – Vol. 66-A. – P. 774–777.

[16] Goddard, H.J. Atlanto-axial rotatory fixation and fracture of the clavicle / H.J. Goddard, J. Stabler, J.S. Albert // J. Bone Joint Surg. – 1990. – Vol. 72-B, N 1. – P. 72–75.

[17] Greeley, P.W. Bilateral (ninety degrees) rotatory dislocation of the atlas upon the axis / P.W. Greeley // J. Bone Joint Surg. – 1930. – Vol. 12. – P. 958–962.

[18] Ono, K. Atlantoaxial rotatory fixation: radiographic study of its mechanism / K. Ono, K. Yonenobu, T. Fuji, K. Okada // Spine. – 1985. – Vol. 10. – P. 602–608.

[19] Schwarz, N. Atlanto-axial rotation and distance in small children. A postmortem study / N. Schwarz, M. Lenz, A. Berzlanovich, W. Smetka // Unfallchir. – 2000. – Vol. 103, N 8. – P. 656–661.

[20] Villas, C. Preliminary CT study of C1-C2 rotational mobility in normal subjects / C. Villas, C. Arriagada, J.L. Zubieta // Eur. Spine J. – 1999. – Vol. 8, N. 3. – P. 223–228.

[21] Vivas, I. Physiological rotatory C1-C2 subluxation in children / I. Vivas, J.L. Zubieta, C. Arriagada, C. Villas // Eur. Radiol. – 1999.- Vol 9 – P. 54.

[22] Fiorani-Gallotta, G. Sublussazione laterale e sublussazione rotatoria dell'atlante / G. Fiorani-Gallotta, G. Luzzatti // Arch. Orthop. – 1957. – Vol. 70, N 5. – P. 467–484.

[23] Maigne, J.Y. Acute torticollis in an adolescent: case report and MRI study / J.Y. Maigne, C. Mutschler, L. Doursounian // Spine. – 2003. – Vol. 28, N 1. – P. 13–15.

[24] Gubin A.V. Etiology of Child Acute Stiff Neck/ Gubin A.V., Ulrich, E.V., Taschilkin, A.I., Yalfimov, A.N.// Spine. - 2009. –Vol.34: pp.1906-1909.

[25] Gubin A.V. «Uncovertebral wedge» as a cause of child's acute stiff-neck./ Gubin A.V., Ulrich, E.V., Taschilkin, A.I., Yalfimov, A.N.// European Journal of Neurology Vol.17, Suppl.3, 2010, p.509

[26] Ellis, G.L. Imaging of the atlas (C1) and axis (C2) / G.L. Ellis // Emerg. Med. Clin. North Am. - 1991. - Vol. 9, N 4. - P. 719–732.
[27] Maheshwaran, S. Imaging of childhood torticollis due to atlanto-axial rotatory fixation / S. Maheshwaran [et al.] // Child's. Nerv. Syst. - 1995. - Vol. 11, N 12. - P. 667–671.
[28] Klein, D.M. Problems in the radiographic diagnosis of atlanto-axial rotation deformity / D.M. Klein, J.P. Kuhn // Conc. Pediat. Neurosurg. - 1985. - Vol. 5. - P. 26–33.
[29] Li, Y.K. Diagnostic value on signs of subluxation of cervical vertebrae with radiological examination / Y.K. Li, Y.K. Zhang, S.Z. Zhong // J. Manipulative Physiol. Ther. - 1998. - Vol. 21, N 9. - P. 617–620.
[30] Lee, S. Asymmetry of the odontoid-lateral mass interspaces: a radiographic finding of questionable clinical significance / S. Lee, S. Joyce, J. Seeger // Ann. Emerg. Med. - 1986. - Vol. 15, N 10. - P. 1173–1176.
[31] Nicholson, P. Three-dimensional spiral CT scanning in children with acute torticollis / P. Nicholson [et al.] // Int. Orthop. - 1999. - Vol. 23, N 1. - P. 47–50.
[32] Fielding, J.W. Atlanto-axial rotatory fixation (fixed rotatory subluxation of the atlanto-axial joint) / J.W. Fielding, R.J. Hawkins // J. Bone Joint Surg. - 1977. - Vol. 59-A. - P. 37–44.
[33] Fielding, J.W. Cineroentgenography of the normal cervical spine / J.W. Fielding // J. Bone Joint Surg. - 1957. - Vol. 39-A. - P. 1280–1288.
[34] Johnson, D.P. Fergusson CM. Early diagnosis of atlantoaxial rotatory fixation / D.P. Johnston // J. Bone Joint. Surg. - 1986. - Vol. 68-B. - P. 698–701.
[35] Rinaldi, I. Computerized tomographic demonstration of rotational atlanto-axial fixation / I. Rinaldi, W.J. Mullins, W.F. Delaney // J. Neurosurg. - 1979. - Vol. 50. - P. 115–119.
[36] Van Hosbeeck, E.M.A. Diagnosis of acute atlanto-axial rotatory fixation / E.M.A. Van Hosbeeck, N.N.S. Mackay // J. Bone Joint Surg. - 1989. - Vol. 71. - P. 90–91.
[37] Dvorak, J. CT-functional diagnostics of the rotatory instability of the upper cervical spine / J. Dvorak, M. Panjabi, M. Gerber, W. Wichmann // Spine. - 1987. - Vol. 12. - P. 197–205.
[38] Li, V. Atlantoaxial rotatory fixation / V. Li, D. Pang // Disorders of the pediatric spine. - New York, 1995. - P. 531–553.
[39] Alanay, A. Reliability and necessity of dynamic computerized tomography in diagnosis of atlantoaxial rotatory subluxation / Alanay A. [et al.] // Spine. - 2002. - Vol. 22, N 6. - P. 763–765.
[40] Hicazi, A. Atlantoaxial rotatory fixation-subluxation revisited: a computed tomographic analysis of acute torticollis in pediatric patients / A. Hicazi [et al.] // Spine. - Vol. 27, N 24. - P. 2771–2775.
[41] Kowalski, H.M. Pitfalls in the CT diagnosis of atlanto-axial rotatory subluxation / H.M. Kowalski, W.A. Cohen, P. Cooper, J.H. Wiscoff // Am. J. Roentgenol. - 1987. - Vol. 149. - P. 595–600.
[42] Park, S.W. Successful reduction for a pediatric chronic atlantoaxial rotatory fixation (Grisel syndrome) with long-term halter traction / Park S.W. [et al.] // Spine. - 2005. - Vol. 30, N 15. - P. 444–449.

[43] Khanna, A.J. Magnetic resonance imaging of the cervical spine: current techniques and spectrum of disease / A.J. Khanna [et al.] // J. Bone Joint Surg. – 2002. – Vol. 84-A. – P. 70–80.

[44] Berkheiser, E.J. Nontraumatic dislocations of the atlanto-axial joint / E.J. Berkheiser, F. Seidler // J. Am. Med. Assn. – 1931. – Vol. 96. – P. 517–523.

[45] Губин А.В. Алгоритм действий хирурга при острой кривошее у детей./ Губин А.В.// Травматология и ортопедия России №1, 2009 с.52-57

Part 5

Spinal Cord Injury

10

Autologous Macrophages Genetically Modified by *Ex Vivo* Electroporation and Inserted by Lumbar Puncture Migrate and Concentrate in Damaged Spinal Cord Tissue: A Safe and Easy Gene Transfer Method for the Treatment of Spinal Cord Injury

Tadanori Ogata, Tadao Morino, Hideki Horiuchi,
Masayuki Hino, Gotaro Yamaoka and Hiromasa Miura
Department of Orthopaedic Surgery, Ehime University School of Medicine
Japan

1. Introduction

Spinal cord injury is one of the most serious conditions in the field of orthopedic surgery. Several pharmacological trials have been performed for the treatment of traumatic spinal cord injury. However, only high-dose steroid therapy has been established as an effective treatment for this condition. It is necessary to develop an effective treatment to inhibit secondary neuronal damage and to promote neuronal regeneration after the spinal cord injury.

Recently, direct delivery of neurotrophic factors, such as nerve growth factor (NGF), glial-derived neurotrophic factor (GDNF), and brain-derived neurotrophic factor (BDNF), has been demonstrated to provide neuroprotection and counteract lesion-induced atrophy after traumatic injury to the central nervous system (CNS) (Kobayashi et al., 1997; Houle et al., 1999; Bregman et al., 2002; Cao et al., 2002; Zhou, et al., 2006).

Intravenous applications of neurotrophic factors, such as GDNF and BDNF, are also possible therapeutic methods. In the injured spinal cord, however, blood flow in the nervous tissue decreases remarkably (Hamamoto et al., 2007). When neuroprotective substances are added intravenously, only a small amount of the substances reach the injured portion of the spinal cord. In addition, the half lives of most proteins in vivo are relatively short. Therefore, systemic intravenous administration of neurotrophic protein may not be an efficient way to treat damaged spinal cord tissue.

Direct infusion of neurotrophic proteins into the neural parenchyma using pumps is another approach to treatment. However, several limitations should be considered as follows: 1) The spread of the proteins throughout the neural parenchyma is often limited. 2) The chronic implantation of the canula in the parenchyma results in the formation of a neural scar at the insertion site. 3) The implanted canula may induce inflammation or clogging of the infusion device. 4) Continuous outflow of liquid can cause additional damage at the insertion site.

Several trials of gene transfer into the CNS have been conducted both *in vivo* and *in vitro*. Adenovirus including the target genes has been successfully used to achieve gene transfer in the CNS (Fink et al., 2000; Miagkov et al., 2004; Kwon et al., 2007). However, viral infection of the CNS may be too dangerous for clinical use because of the risk of meningitis (Driesse et al., 2000).

To develop a novel system for substance delivery to damaged ischemic tissue, we focused on the tissue-migration ability of macrophages. Macrophages migrate into damaged tissue or inflammatory tissue. After spinal cord injury, the appearance of macrophages in the damaged tissue has been reported (Dusart et al., 1994; Morino et al., 2003). For this study, gene transfer by *ex vivo* electroporation, a non-viral gene transfer method, was performed on autologous macrophages, and the cells were injected into the subarachnoid space. It is believed that if the cells migrate and concentrate in the damaged spinal cord, it will provide a safe and effective method of substance delivery to the damaged spinal cord parenchyma.

2. Experimental procedures

2.1 Animals

A total of 56 male Wistar rats (350 g-weight, purchased from Japan Clea Co., Japan) were used for this experiment (in vivo 50, in vitro 6). The research protocol was accepted by the ethical committee for animal experiments at Ehime University (Ehime, Japan).

2.2 Collection of autologous macrophages and GFP gene incorporation

Intraperitoneal macrophages were easily collected from rats. The intraperitoneal space was rinsed with 30 ml of Dulbecco's modified Eagle medium (DMEM, Gibco, Grand Island, NY) via midline incision of the abdomen. The DMEM, which contained a large concentration of macrophages, was collected and centrifuged, and cells were re-suspended in cell permeabilization buffer (140 mM KCl, 5 mM NaCl, 10 mM glucose, 0.5 mM EGTA, 10 mM HEPES, pH 7.2). To identify gene-transfected cells, we used pEGFPLuc Vector (Clontech Inc. USA). This vector was constructed by inserting the GFP gene for over-expression of GFP protein. 200 μl of the cells (1×10^6 cells /ml) were mixed with 20 μl of GFP-containing vector in disposable cuvette-electrodes (2 mm gap, BTZ 620, BTX Inc., USA). The final concentration of the vector was 0.1 μg/μl. Then, six 20 ms electric pulses of 20 V were applied by electroporator (CUY 21, NEPA GENE Co., Japan). The treated cells were then cultured (*in vitro*) or returned to the animals by intrathecal application (*in vivo*).

2.3 Cell culturing and observation of GFP protein expression

The gene-transfected macrophages were cultured in 6-well culture plates (Nunc, Naperville, IL) at a concentration of 5×10^4 cells/well with DMEM containing 15% fetal calf serum. Culturing was performed in a humidified 5% CO_2 atmosphere at 37°C. Seven days after culturing, the cells were observed under a fluorescent microscope.

2.4 Spinal cord injury model (SCI model)

Under general anesthesia using halothane, the rat spinal cord was carefully exposed by removing the vertebral lamina at the 11th vertebra. Spinal cord impact injury was performed using a MASCIS Impactor (New Jersey, USA). The impact weight was dropped from a height of 25 mm. In one group of rats, a laminectomy of the 11th vertebra was performed without spinal cord injury (sham).

2.5 Macrophage transplantation into the spinal cord by lumbar puncture

100 μl of a liquid suspension of the gene-transfected macrophages (1×10^5 cells) was injected into the subarachnoid space at the $4\text{-}5^{th}$ lumbar intervertebral level just after the spinal cord injury.

2.6 Histological examination

Rats were sacrificed for histological study by deep anesthesia using diethyl ether and their spinal cords were taken out immediately. Horizontal or axial frozen sections with a thickness of 20 μm were produced, and autofluorescence was observed under fluorescence microscopy. To quantify the number of migrated gene-transfected macrophages, photographs at an area peripheral to the center of the SCI were taken and the number of GFP-positive cells were counted by three individuals who did not know any information about the pictures. For the first 96 hours after the SCI, the GFP autofluorescence was weak, and therefore, the cells were hardly distinguishable from the background until after 96 hours had elapsed. The counts were averaged and data were expressed as the number of GFP-positive cells per 1 mm^2.

To confirm the expression of transferred GFP, some sections were subjected to immunostaining by anti-GFP antibody according to avidin-biotin-complex (ABC) method using Vectastain ABC kit (Vector labo. Inc., CA). The sections were fixed on glass slides with 4% paraformaldehyde in phosphate-buffered saline (PBS) for 5 minutes. Then, after washing twice with PBS, endogenous peroxidase was blocked by treatment with 3% H_2O_2/H_2O for 5 minutes. Slices were exposed to anti-GFP antibody (1:1000 in 1% horse serum/PBS; MBL Co., Ltd., Nagoya, Japan) overnight at 4°C. Sections were then washed by PBS and exposed to biotin-conjugated anti-rabbit IgG for 1 hour at room temperature. After washing the antibody, sections were treated by ABC method according to the assay protocol of the kit, and finally colour developed with 3,3'-diaminobenzidine tetrahydrochloride (DAB, Wako Chemicals Ltd.) substrate (0.02% H_2O_2 plus 0.1% DAB in 0.1M Tris-buffer) for 5 minutes and washed immediately with water for 20 minutes. Sections were dehydrated through graded alcohols and xylene and were then mounted in HSR solution (Yoshitomi co., Osaka, Japan).

To clarify which kinds of cells had been transplanted, some sections were subjected to immunostaining by OX-42, a marker of macrophages. Frozen sections were prepared according to the method mentioned above. Then, after washing twice with PBS, slices on slides were exposed to anti-OX42 antibody (Immunotech. Co. Marseille, France) overnight at 4°C, and rhodamine-conjugated anti-mouse IgG antibody (Chemicon International Co. CA, USA) for 1 hour. The sections were then observed under fluorescent microscopy.

2.7 Evaluation of motor function

Motor function was assessed with the Basso, Beattie and Bresnahan (BBB) scoring scale (Basso et al., 1996). The BBB scale is a 21-point scale that ranks no locomotion as 0 points and a normal gait as 21 points. The BBB scale is one of the most widely used methods for evaluating hind-limb motor function in rats and mice. Hind-limb motor function was evaluated at 2, 3, 4, 7, 14, 21, 28, and 56 days after SCI. The evaluation of BBB scores was done by three individuals who were unaware of the treatments that the rats had received. The average of the three observers' scores was employed as data in this study.

3. Results

3.1 Expression of green fluorescent protein (GFP) protein in cultured gene-transfected macrophages

The cultured cells were observed under fluorescent microscopy. Detectable autofluorescence was observed from the 3rd day of the culture, and the intensity of the autofluorescence increased with time. Fig 1 shows an example of typical autofluorescence at 7 days after culturing. We were able to maintain cells with autofluorescence in a culture dish for 2 weeks.

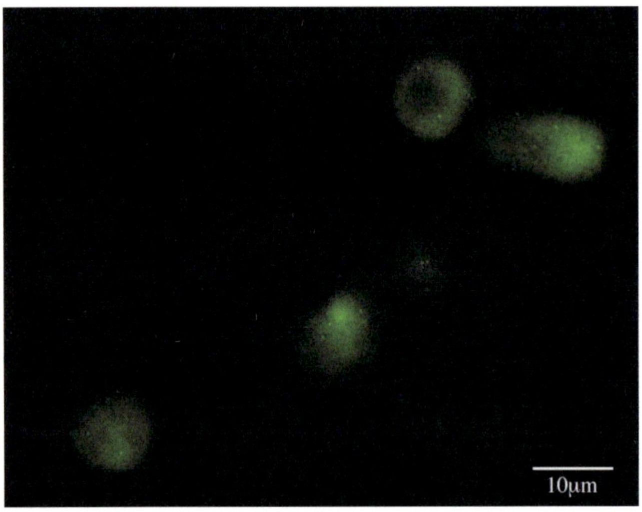

Fig. 1. Photographs of typical GFP autofluorescence in cultured macrophages 7 days after culturing.

Intra-peritoneal macrophages were harvested from a rat. Then vectors containing GFP were transferred by ex vivo electroporation.

3.2 Hind-limb motor function after spinal cord injuries (SCI)

In sham animals, those without an impact injury, no symptoms were observed in the lower limbs (21 points). In the rats with spinal cord injuries (SCI), almost complete paresis of the hind limbs was observed just after the injury (0 points). Motor function recovery started 7 days after the injury, and the recovery reached a plateau at 4 weeks after the injury (13.7 ±

0.94 points). The paresis did not recover until 8 weeks after the injury (Fig. 2). BBB scores in the sham animals were consistently 21 points.

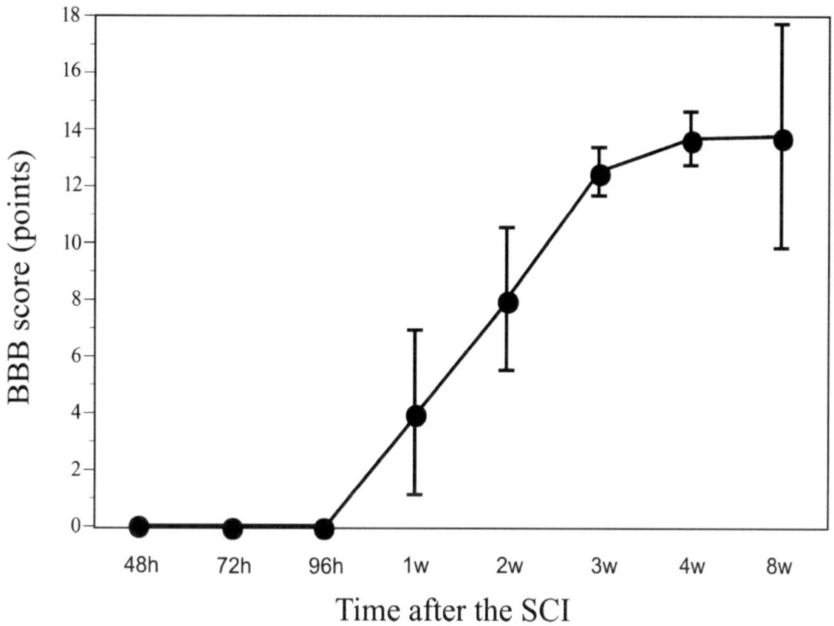

Fig. 2. Time course of hind-limb motor function after spinal cord injury evaluated by the BBB scale.

Spinal cord impact injury was performed using a MASCIS impactor. The impact weight was dropped from a height of 25 mm. Hind-limb motor function was evaluated using the BBB scale. Data are mean ± SEM (n = 4 to 6).

3.3 Histological results

In slices obtained from SCI rats three or four days after the injury, weak autofluorescence was detected in the center of the compressed part and on the surface of the spinal cord (data not shown). One week after the injury, the fluorescence was strong enough to easily differentiate between fluorescent and non-fluorescent cells. From this point, we were able to count the number of GFP-positive cells in the slices.

Injected macrophages migrated and concentrated in the injured part of the spinal cord. Most of the GFP-positive cells were detected in the gray matter, especially in the area peripheral to the cavity caused by necrotic cell death (Fig. 3A). There were few GFP-positive cells in the white matter or the pia mater (Fig. 3B). There were few GFP-positive cells in the areas 1-cm rostral or caudal to the center of impact (data not shown). In summary, most of the GFP-positive cells appeared in the injured area in spite of the fact that the cells were injected intrathecally. This result indicates that the injected autologous macrophages migrated and concentrated in the gray matter of the injured spinal cord.

Fluorescence intensity and the number of GFP-positive cells increased with time and peaked at three weeks after the injury (Fig. 4). Figure 5 shows the time course of the number of countable GFP-positive cells. The number of GFP-positive cells peaked at three weeks after the SCI (32.0 ± 10.3 cells / mm^2 in 20 μm slice). Autofluorescence was detected even 2 months after the injury/injection. The gene-transfected macrophages successfully stayed in the injured area and survived for a long period of time.

In order to confirm that autofluorescence was detected only from GFP gene-transfected macrophages, we performed anti-GFP staining (Fig. 6) and OX-42 staining (Fig. 7) in slices obtained two weeks after the injury.

Figure 6 shows anti-GFP staining of the thoracic spinal cord. The cells, which were positive to anti-GFP antibody, were observed in the thoracic spinal cord tissue in the area peripheral to the cavity caused by necrotic cell death.

OX-42 staining (Fig. 7) showed that most of the OX-42-positive macrophages revealed GFP autofluorescence. There were a few OX-42-positive cells which did not show autofluorescence. These cells might be microglia which appeared after the injury. All of the GFP-positive cells were also positive for OX-42.

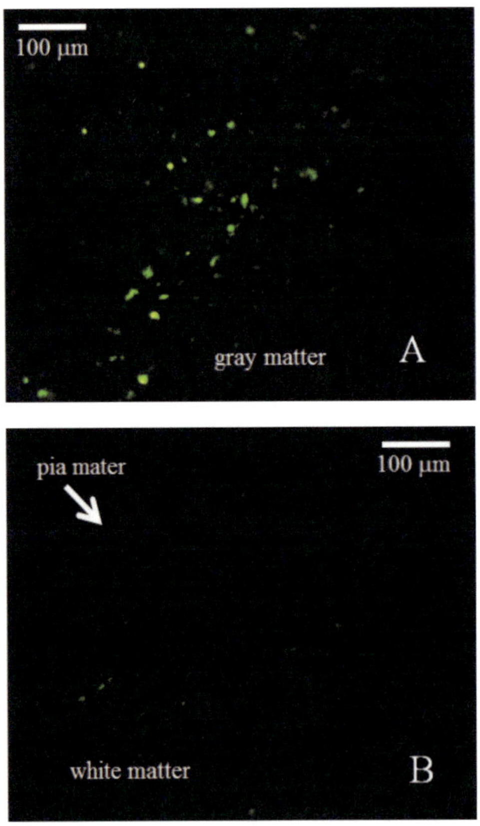

Fig. 3. Distribution of GFP-positive macrophages in the spinal cord four weeks after transplantation.

GFP-gene transfected autologous macrophages were injected by lumbar puncture after the spinal cord injury. Four weeks after the injection, a sample of the injured spinal cord was taken and axial sections were subjected to histological examination. Most of the GFP-positive cells were detected in the gray matter (A). There were few GFP-positive cells in the white matter or in the pia mater (B).

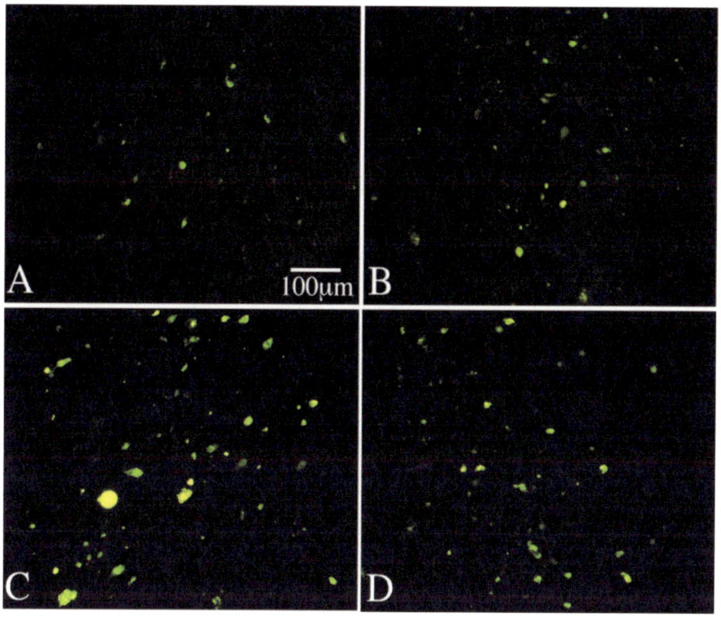

Fig. 4. Autofluorescence of GFP-positive macrophages in the gray matter of the injured spinal cord. GFP-gene transfected autologous macrophages were injected by lumbar puncture after the spinal cord injury. One (A), two (B), three (C) and four (D) weeks after the injury/injection, a sample of the injured spinal cord was taken and horizontal sections were subjected to histological examination. The pictures show the areas peripheral to the center of the impact injury.

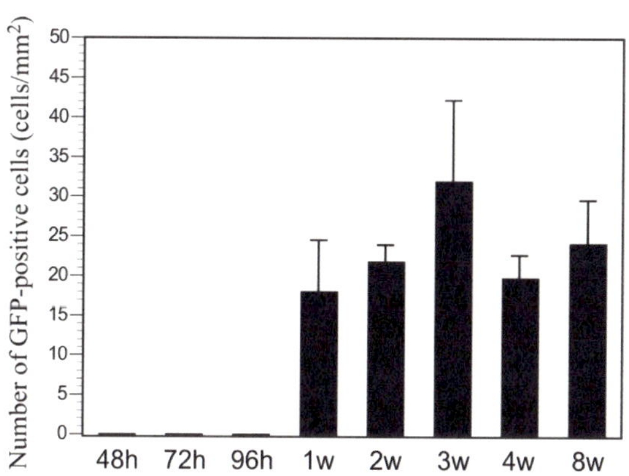

Fig. 5. Number of GFP-positive cells in the center of the damaged spinal cord tissue.

At the indicated time point after the injury/injection, a sample of the injured spinal cord was taken and horizontal sections were subjected to histological examination. The cells, which revealed significant autofluorescence in the area peripheral to the center of impact injury, were counted. Data are shown in mean ± SEM (n = 4 to 6).

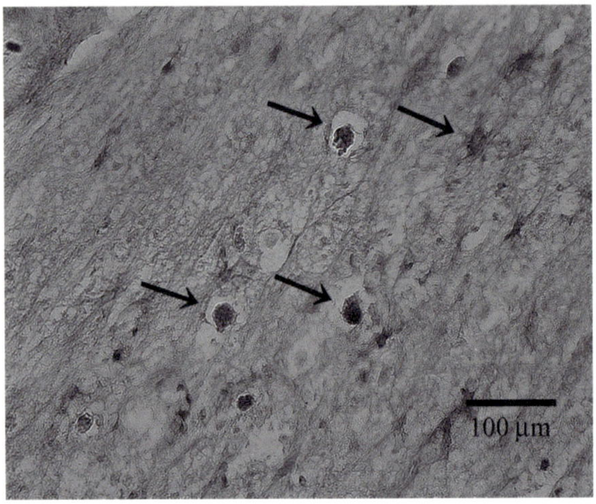

Fig. 6. Anti-GFP staining of the spinal cord two weeks after transplantation.

Two weeks after the injection, a sample of the injured spinal cord was taken and horizontal sections were subjected to histological examination. Horizontal sections in the thoracic spinal cord were stained by anti-GFP antibody. Gene-transferred autologous macrophages migrated into the spinal cord tissue (arrows).

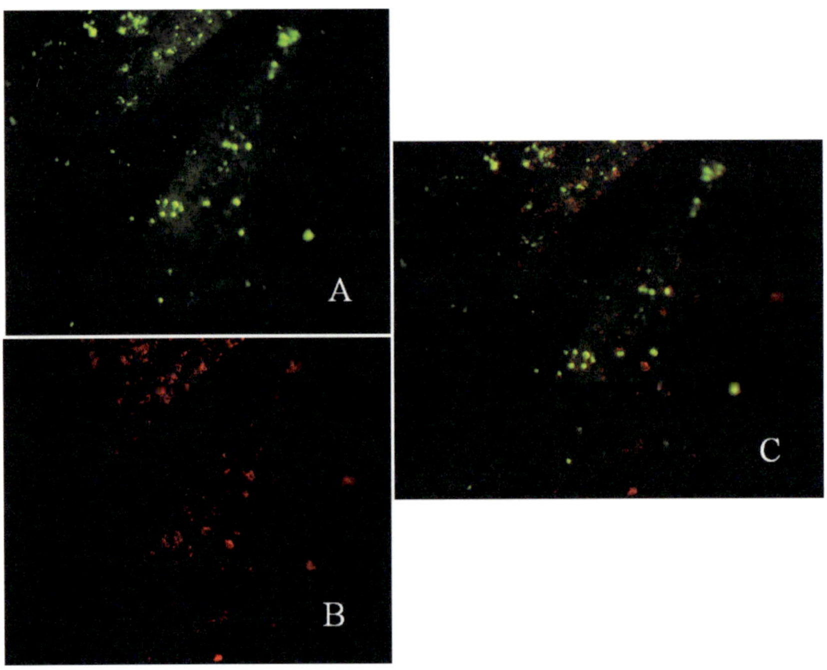

Fig. 7. Co-localization of OX-42 and GFP protein in the cells in the injured portion of spinal cord.

Two weeks after the injection, a sample of the injured spinal cord was taken and horizontal sections were subjected to histological examination. A: autofluorescence of GFP-positive cells, B: OX-42 immunoreactive cells, C: Overlap photograph of GFP autofluorescence and OX-42. Most of the OX-42-positive macrophages showed GFP autofluorescence.

4. Discussion

Gene transfer to injured spinal cord tissue is thought to be an effective method for the treatment of spinal cord injury. For example, over-expression of neurotrophic factors, such as NGF or BDNF, may be an effective method of promoting the recovery of motor function, and over-expression of endogenous opioids, such as endorphin or enkephalin, may be effective for the reduction of hyperalgesia or spontaneous pain after spinal cord injury.

Electroporation has been used for several types of gene transfer, such as muscle (Watanabe et al., 2001), skin (Maruyama et al., 2001), tumor (Yamashita et al., 2001), and spinal cord gene transfer (Lin et al., 2002). To establish a method of transferring the gene into macrophages, we tested electroporation under several different conditions. Technical procedures for electroporation have been reported, but considerable variation in the ideal intensity of electric stimulation has been described in the literature. Since no report describing a method of electroporation for macrophages was available, we have tested several conditions to determine a proper method to treat macrophages. In particular, the stimulation voltage and duration were very important. When we applied six 20 ms pulses of 20 V to the cuvette-electrode with a 2 mm gap, the total current was between 1.1 and 1.4 A. More than 80% of the surviving macrophages showed autofluorescence in the culture plate (data not shown). When we applied a voltage higher than 50V or applied a pulse for a duration longer than 50 ms, most of the cells died within 48 hours. When we applied six 20 ms pulse of 10 V, the cells survived, but no detectable autofluorescence was seen within 1 week. Therefore, we think the conditions we used in this study are ideal for macrophage electroporation.

Direct implantation of several kinds of cells into the damaged spinal cord has been reported. These reports show that implantation of several kinds of cells into the damaged nervous tissue may promote neuronal regeneration. The candidates for donor cells for spinal cord injuries are bone marrow stromal cells (Kamada et al., 2005), macrophages (Rapalino et al., 1998; Schwartz et al., 1999) and neural stem cells (Iwanami et al., 2005). However, direct injection of the cells into the spinal cord may be a dangerous procedure for clinical use. Recently, more less-invasive transplantation procedures have been reported. Bakshi et al.(2004, 2006) reported that bone marrow stem cells and neural precursor cells migrated into the damaged spinal cord tissue via intrathecal injection. Lepore et al. (2005) also reported that neural stem cells migrated into the damaged spinal cord tissue via intrathecal injection. They also tested the intravenous injection of neural stem cells. Some stem cells reached the damaged spinal cord tissue, although not as many as in the intrathecal injection procedure. In our result, the intrathecally injected autologous macrophage appeared around the center of damaged spinal cord tissue. There were few migrated macrophage in the areas 1-cm rostral or caudal to the center of impact. These results suggest that the cells, which have migration activity similar to immature stem cells, are led to the damaged tissue.

Macrophages, immune cells which are distributed widely in the body, have strong migratory abilities. In the vessels, they usually exist as monocytes. There are about 4 x 10^8

cells per 1 liter of blood. When inflammation occurs, they migrate into the damaged tissue and change into macrophages. Macrophages are available in injured nervous tissue after spinal cord or peripheral nerve injuries (Leskovar et al., 2000; Morino et al., 2003). Inflammation after an injury may be an inducer of monocyte/macrophage migration. The hypothesis of this study was that if autologous macrophages exist in the subarachnoid space after a spinal cord injury, they may migrate and concentrate in the center of the inflamed or damaged area. This hypothesis has proven to be correct. In the present study, macrophages were collected from rats, and plasmids including the target gene were transferred into the cells by *ex vivo* electroporation. Then, the gene-transfected autologous macrophages were returned to the subarachnoid space. We successfully implanted the gene-transfected autologous macrophages into the injured part of the spinal cord by intrathecal injection. This method is much safer than direct injection of the cells into the injured area.

Neuroprotective therapies using neurotrophic factors may be effective not only for acute spinal cord injuries, but also for chronic stages after the injury. Kwon et al. (2002) reported that rubrospinal neurons, whose axons had been cut in the cervical spinal cord 1 year before, have regenerative capacity and that massive atrophy of rubrospinal neurons can be reversed by applying BDNF.

Therefore, we should develop therapeutic methods for the treatment of both the acute and chronic phase of the neurodegenerative and regenerative processes. For the treatment of the acute phase of spinal cord injury, we previously reported that hypothermic treatment (Ogata et al., 2000) and intrathecal application of SB203580, a selective inhibitor of p38 mitogen-activated protein kinase (Horiuchi et al., 2003) effectively induced motor function recovery after SCI. For treatment of more chronic stages of SCI, continuous delivery of neuroprotective or neuroregenerative substances, such as neurotrophic proteins, should be required for at least several months. In the present study, we demonstrated that implanted autologous macrophages survived for a long period of time (more than 2 months) and GFP expression continued from one week to 2 months after the injection (Fig. 5). If this procedure of gene transfer by a single injection is performed every two months, substance delivery can be achieved continuously for one year or more.

Since an enormous amount of intra-peritoneal macrophages can be easily collected from rats or mice, we used intra-peritoneal macrophages in the present study. If this procedure is used in humans, monocytes, the precursor cells of macrophages, could be collected from peripheral blood and used instead of macrophages. Since a considerable amount of monocytes can be easily collected from peripheral blood, repetitive cell transplantation via lumbar puncture may be carried out easily.

In summary, we successfully transferred the GFP gene into the damaged spinal cord via gene-transfected autologous macrophages by intrathecal injection. This method may be a useful substance-delivery system for the treatment of spinal cord injury.

5. Conclusion

In the present study, we successfully transferred the GFP gene into the damaged spinal cord via gene-transfected autologous macrophages by intrathecal injection. This method may be a useful substance-delivery system for the treatment of spinal cord injury.

6. References

Bakshi, A., Barshinger, A.L., Swanger, S.A., Madhavani, V., Shumsky, J.S., Neuhuber, B. & Fischer, I. (2006). Lumbar puncture delivery of bone marrow stromal cells in spinal cord contusion: a novel method for minimally invasive cell transplantation. *J Neurotrauma*. 23: 55-65.

Bakshi, A., Hunter, C., Swanger, S., Lepore, A. & Fischer, I. (2004) Minimally invasive delivery of stem cells for spinal cord injury: advantages of the lumbar puncture technique. J. Neurosurg. *Spine* 1: 330-337.

Basso, D.M., Beattie, M.S. & Bresnahan, J.C. (1996) Graded histological and locomotor outcomes after spinal cord contusion using the NYU weight-drop device versus transection. *Exp. Neurol.* 139: 244-256

Bregman, B.S., Coumans, J.V., Dai, H.N., Kuhn, P.L., Lynskey, J., McAtee, M. & Sandhu, F. (2002) Transplants and neurotrophic factors increase regeneration and recovery of function after spinal cord injury. *Prog. Brain Res.* 137: 257-273.

Cao, X., Tang, C. & Luo, Y. (2002) Effect of nerve growth factor on neuronal apoptosis after spinal cord injury in rats. *Chin. J. Traumatol.* 5: 131-135.

Driesse, M.J., Esandi, M.C., Kros, J.M., Avezaat, C.J., Vecht, C., Zurcher, C., van der Velde, I., Valerio, D., Bout, A. & Sillevis Smitt, P.A. (2000) Intra-CSF administered recombinant adenovirus causes an immune response-mediated toxicity. *Gene Ther.* 7: 1401-1409.

Dusart, I. & Schwab, M.E. (1994) Secondary cell death and the inflammatory reaction after dorsal hemisection of the rat spinal cord. *Eur. J. Neurosci.* 6: 712-724.

Fink, S.L., Ho, D.Y., McLaughlin, J. & Sapolsky, R.M. (2000) An adenoviral vector expressing the glucose transporter protects cultured striatal neurons from 3-nitropropionic acid. *Brain Res.* 859:21-25.

Hamamoto, Y., Ogata, T., Morino, T., Hino, M. & Yamamoto, H. (2007) Real-time direct measurement of spinal cord blood flow at the site of compression: relationship between blood flow recovery and motor deficiency in spinal cord injury. *Spine* 32: 1955-1962.

Horiuchi, H., Ogata, T., Morino, T., Chuai, M. & Yamamoto, H. (2003) Continuous intrathecal infusion of SB203580, a selective inhibitor of p38 mitogen-activated protein kinase, reduces the damage of hind-limb function after thoracic spinal cord injury in rat. *Neurosci. Res.* 47: 209-217.

Houle, J.D. & Ye, J.H. (1999) Survival of chronically-injured neurons can be prolonged by treatment with neurotrophic factors. *Neuroscience* 94: 929-936.

Iwanami, A., Kaneko, S., Nakamura, M., Kanemura, Y., Mori, H., Kobayashi, S., Yamasaki, M., Momoshima, S., Ishii, H., Ando, K., Tanioka, Y., Tamaoki, N., Nomura, T., Toyama, Y. & Okano, H. (2005) Transplantation of human neural stem cells for spinal cord injury in primates. *J. Neurosci. Res.* 80: 182-190.

Kamada, T., Koda, M., Dezawa, M., Yoshinaga, K., Hashimoto, M., Koshizuka, S., Nishio, Y., Moriya, H. & Yamazaki, M. (2005) Transplantation of bone marrow stromal cell-derived Schwann cells promotes axonal regeneration and functional recovery after complete transection of adult rat spinal cord. *J Neuropathol. Exp. Neurol.* 64: 37-45.

Kobayashi, N.R., Fan, D.P., Giehl, K.M., Bedard, A.M., Wiegand, S.J. & Tetzlaff, W. (1997) BDNF and NT-4/5 prevent atrophy of rat rubrospinal neurons after cervical axotomy, stimulate GAP-43 and Talpha1-tubulin mRNA expression, and promote axonal regeneration. *J. Neurosci.* 17: 9583-9595.

Kwon, B.K., Liu, J., Lam, C., Plunet, W., Oschipok, L.W., Hauswirth, W., Di Polo, A., Blesch, A. & Tetzlaff, W. (2007) Brain-derived neurotrophic factor gene transfer with adeno-associated viral and lentiviral vectors prevents rubrospinal neuronal atrophy and stimulates regeneration-associated gene expression after acute cervical spinal cord injury. *Spine* 32: 1164-1173.

Kwon, B.K., Liu, J., Messerer, C., Kobayashi, N.R., McGraw, J., Oschipok, L. & Tetzlaff, W. (2002) Survival and regeneration of rubrospinal neurons 1 year after spinal cord injury. *Proc. Natl. Acad. Sci. U S A.* 99: 3246-3251.

Lepore, A.C., Bakshi, A., Swanger, S.A., Rao, M.S. & Fischer, I. (2005) Neural precursor cells can be delivered into the injured cervical spinal cord by intrathecal injection at the lumbar cord. *Brain Res.* 1045: 206-216.

Leskovar, A., Moriarty, L.J., Turek, J.J., Schoenlein, I.A. & Borgens, R.B. (2000) The macrophage in acute neural injury: changes in cell numbers over time and levels of cytokine production in mammalian central and peripheral nervous systems. *J. Exp. Biol.* 203: 1783-1795.

Lin, C.R., Tai, M.H., Cheng, J.T., Chou, A.K., Wang, J.J., Tan, P.H., Marsala, M. & Yang, L.C. (2002) Electroporation for direct spinal gene transfer in rats. *Neurosci. Lett.* 317: 1-4.

Maruyama, H., Ataka, K., Higuchi, N., Sakamoto, F., Gejyo, F. & Miyazaki, J. (2001) Skin-targeted gene transfer using in vivo electroporation. *Gene Ther.* 8: 1808-1812.

Miagkov, A., Turchan, J., Nath, A. & Drachman, D.B. (2004) Gene transfer of baculoviral p35 by adenoviral vector protects human cerebral neurons from apoptosis. *DNA Cell Biol.* 23: 496-501.

Morino, T., Ogata, T., Horiuchi, H., Takeba, J., Okumura, H., Miyazaki, T. & Yamamoto, H. (2003) Delayed neuronal damage related to microglia proliferation after mild spinal cord compression injury. *Neurosci. Res.* 46: 309-318.

Ogata, T., Morino, T., Takeba, J., Matsuda, Y., Okumura, H., Shibata, T., Schubert, P. & Kataoka, K. (2000) Mild hypothermia amelioration of damage during rat spinal cord injury: inhibition of pathological microglial proliferation and improvement of hind-limb motor function, in Hayashi N (ed.), *Brain Hypothermia*, Springer-Verlag, Tokyo, pp. 47-54.

Rapalino, O., Lazarov-Spiegler, O., Agranov, E., Velan, G.J., Yoles, E., Fraidakis, M., Solomon, A., Gepstein, R., Katz, A., Belkin, M., Hadani, M. & Schwartz, M. (1998). Implantation of stimulated homologous macrophages results in partial recovery of paraplegic rats. *Nat. Med.* 4: 814-821.

Schwartz, M., Lazarov-Spiegler, O., Rapalino, O., Agranov, I., Velan, G. & Hadani, M. (1999) Potential repair of rat spinal cord injuries using stimulated homologous macrophages. *Neurosurg.* 44: 1041-1045.

Watanabe, K., Nakazawa, M., Fuse, K., Hanawa, H., Kodama, M., Aizawa, Y., Ohnuki, T., Gejyo, F., Maruyama, H. & Miyazaki, J. (2001) Protection against autoimmune myocarditis by gene transfer of interleukin-10 by electroporation. *Circulation* 104: 1098-1100.

Yamashita, Y.I., Shimada, M., Hasegawa, H., Minagawa, R., Rikimaru, T., Hamatsu, T., Tanaka, S., Shirabe, K., Miyazaki, J.I. & Sugimachi, K. (2001) Electroporation-mediated interleukin-12 gene therapy for hepatocellular carcinoma in the mice model. *Cancer Res.* 61: 1005-1012.

Zhou, L.H. & Wu, W. (2006) Survival of injured spinal motoneurons in adult rat upon treatment with glial cell line-derived neurotrophic factor at 2 weeks but not at 4 weeks after root avulsion. *J. Neurotrauma* 23: 920-927.